Mechanical Ventilation for the ICU Resident

Copyright © 2021

Rafiq Kutty MD

ISBN 9798789109403

Mechanical Ventilation for the ICU Resident

A Concept Based Approach

R Kutty MD FCCP

Preface

This book is written primarily with the intent of helping medical residents understand the basics of mechanical ventilation. It is meant to be read during a one-month rotation in the ICU. It is not a comprehensive text. It also presupposes a certain amount of background medical knowledge that most residents in training should have. It is a compilation of concepts and explanations that were formed during teaching rounds in the ICU, at St. Francis Hospital in Evanston, IL. As residents and students would ask questions regarding the ventilator, I was compelled to answer those questions in a manner that was practical for the resident. As a result, the content herein is somewhat unique, in that it was developed in response to those questions, and is therefore tailored to the needs of residents in training. Most medicine residents want to know about the ventilator more than anything else while in the ICU. After being asked which ventilator resource would be most helpful many times, and not being able to give a very good answer, I decided to write this little book.

Acknowledgements

I would like to acknowledge the residents on service whose questions formulated the basis of this book. I would also like to acknowledge my wife, who helped with formatting of the text.

Contents

1. Indications for Mechanical Ventilation 1
2. Ventilator Parameters 3
3. Modes of Ventilation 8
4. Respiratory Mechanics and Concepts 18
5. Ventilation in Specific Circumstances... 32
6. Liberation from Mechanical Ventilation.. 35
7. Advanced Oxygenation Techniques 42
8. Sedatives for Mechanical Ventilation.. 45
9. Neuromuscular Blockade 47
10. Estimating the Degree of Lung Injury 50
11. Complications of Mechanical Ventilation.. 52
12. Other Modes of Oxygenation/Ventilation.. 55
13. Practical Respiratory Physiology... 58
14. Illustrative Cases 65
15. Acid Base Chart... 75

vi

1. Indications for Mechanical Ventilation

The main indications for mechanical ventilation are: hypoxemic respiratory failure, hypercapnic respiratory failure, non-sustainable work of breathing and airway protection. Also, many times, a patient will have a multifactorial problem that necessitates ventilation. For example, very septic patients oftentimes are lethargic due to encephalopathy, and have marginal airway protection. They may be hypoxemic, acidotic and have metabolic derangements as well. Each problem by itself may not warrant intubation, but the totality of problems many times will warrant it. This brings us to our first CONCEPT: The decision to intubate a patient is based on a holistic assessment of the patient, and not on any single parameter. If a dialysis patient is in pulmonary edema, and requires 100% BI-level NIV, then administering stat dialysis may correct the problem and avoid an intubation. If a patient with pneumonia/ARDS is on 100% Bi-level NIV, the natural history of this disease process tells us this is not rapidly correctable, and thus the patient very likely would require intubation and ventilation. A patient on a nonrebreather mask who is awake, alert, and talking, may not require intubation, whereas a patient on a nonrebreather who is poorly responsive, may.

The ventilator has many salutary effects that allow it to facilitate treatment of respiratory failure. Firstly, it is very effective at delivering oxygen. The ventilator can deliver 100% FiO2 and 20cm H20 of PEEP. Bi-level noninvasive ventilation (Bipap®) set at 100% FiO2 can also deliver a fair amount of oxygen. However, the ventilator is superior due to a multitude of reasons. It does not suffer from mask leaks. Patient comfort and tolerability is less of an issue because heavy sedation can be administered. Patients can be fed easily via an NG tube, whereas on Bi-level NIV this can be difficult. Patients can also be transported easier while on the ventilator. Advanced modes of oxygenation can be employed such as prone ventilation, NM blockade, and Nitric Oxide. The tidal volume delivered can be controlled more accurately while on the ventilator. Acid-base balance can be managed better, as one can control PCO2 to a greater degree on a ventilator.

The ventilator offloads work of breathing well. It can entirely replace the respiratory demands of the patient. The inflated cuff of the endotracheal tube can provide protection from large volume aspiration events, and also recurrent small volume aspiration as well.

Initial ventilator settings after intubation are commonly: rate of 12, tidal volume of 500, FiO2 of 100% and PEEP of 5. Some common sense needs to be used here. If the patient's respiratory rate was 40 prior to intubation, very likely they will need a RR greater than 12 when on the ventilator. So, modify the initial settings according to your judgment. Half an hour or so after the patient is intubated, and is in a stable state on the ventilator and sedated, a blood gas should be drawn, and tidal volume, RR and FiO2 can be adjusted accordingly.

When placing the patient on the ventilator, one needs to reflect on why this is needed. If the reason is hypoxemia, then the patient will require a high FiO2 and PEEP. If the reason is work of breathing or tachypnea, then a high RR may be needed to keep up with the patient's ventilatory requirement. If the reason is for airway protection, then only minimal ventilator settings may be required.

2. Ventilator Parameters

In this chapter, we will describe what each parameter on the ventilator is. Looking at all the information provided on the main screen of the ventilator may be daunting. It is useful to start by understanding that the ventilator displays both *set* and *measured* parameters. These are usually displayed on two different locations on the screen. On the Puritan Bennett 840, the measured parameters are on the top of the screen and the set parameters are on the bottom. When we refer to measured parameters, we are referring to measurements the ventilator takes based on the returned air from the patient. The set parameters are parameters set by the physician or RT. Take a moment to familiarize yourself with the layout of the screen on the ventilators used at your facility.

<u>Peak Pressure (Ppeak)</u>
This is the highest pressure recorded during a breath. It is a function of both airway resistance and lung compliance. Many other factors can also contribute to the peak pressure. Learning how to troubleshoot the peak pressure alarm is very important, as it is the most common ventilator alarm to go off. The alarm limit is set by the RT, and is usually around 50cm H20. Generally speaking, a peak pressure of < 30cm H20 is acceptable. If it is higher than that, one may need to investigate why. In many cases, however, it is just a result of a stiff and damaged lung. There are patient factors and ventilator factors that can set off the peak pressure alarm.

A) Patient factors

Poor lung compliance as seen in pulmonary fibrosis, ARDS, pulmonary edema etc., can increase peak pressure because it takes more pressure to fill a stiff lung. Pneumothorax, atelectasis of a lobe or lung, and right main stem intubation can increase peak pressure due to a loss of lung volume. Increased airway resistance as seen in COPD, asthma, and bronchoconstriction, can also increase peak airway pressure by making it difficult for air to flow into the lung. Autopeep can increase peak airway pressure by hyperinflating the lung to a stiffer point on the compliance curve. Coughing and poor ventilator synchrony will commonly increase peak airway pressures.

B) Ventilator and Circuit factors

When the peak pressure alarm goes off, do not automatically think there is something wrong with the patient. High set tidal volumes can increase Ppeak, as more pressure is required to fill the lung with more air. High ventilator flow rates or a square waveform flow pattern can increase Ppeak, as can be ascertained from the equation: Pressure = Flow x Resistance. High levels of PEEP may increase the Ppeak. Mucus secretions in the endotracheal tube will increase Ppeak. If the suction cannula is not fully retracted, and is left partially sitting in the endotracheal tube, the Ppeak will be elevated. This has occurred many times. If the patient is biting on the endotracheal tube, the Ppeak will rise. There is a device on many ventilator circuits called the 'Heat and Moisture Exchanger' or HME (Fig 8). This device functions as a vapor trap, and traps moisture on the patient side of the circuit, thereby moisturizing the inspired air. If this device gets saturated with secretions, the Ppeak will rise. If you suspect this, have RT change the HME. In my personal experience, secretions in the endotracheal tube are the most common cause of a peak pressure alarm going off, so probably the first thing you should do if this happens is suction the patient.

Mean airway pressure (Pmean)
This is the mean pressure measured during both inspiration and expiration, and includes the time spent in between breaths. This means that if you increase the respiratory rate, the mean pressure will go up, as more time will be spent at the higher pressures during the breath and less time spent at the lower pressure between breaths. On the surface of it, Pmean seems like a great parameter to titrate ventilator settings to in order to minimize lung injury, but surprisingly, most of the data targets Pplat and Dp (discussed later) rather than Pmean.

Respiratory rate (RR) or f
This is the respiratory rate in breaths per minute. Sometimes abbreviated 'f' for frequency.

Tidal volume (Vt)
Tidal volume. The volume delivered during a breath.

Minute ventilation (VE)
Minute ventilation. The amount of air expired (or inspired) from the lung in one minute. Units is Liters/min (lpm). Generally speaking, 5-15 lpm is acceptable. Minute ventilation is a good indicator of the patient's ventilatory requirement or work of breathing.

Flow (V̇)
This is the flow rate in lpm the ventilator is delivering the breath at. Commonly it is set at 60 lpm. The common range is 50-90 lpm. The abbreviation is the letter V with a period in the middle of it.

Flow pattern
There is a button on the ventilator with a graphic that looks like a shark fin. This is the flow pattern. It can be set as a decelerating pattern 'shark fin', or as a square wave. The decelerating pattern starts high and decelerates. If you set the flow

rate at 60 lpm, it would start delivering the breath at 60 lpm and then taper off. This is readily seen on the flow tracing on the ventilator screen (Fig 1). The square wave pattern does not decelerate or taper. If you set the flow rate at 60 lpm, it would start at 60 lpm and continue at 60 lpm until the breath was finished. This means it is forcing air into the lung faster. Consequently, the peak pressure goes up, while the inspiratory time (I-time) and mean pressure drop. The mean pressure drops because it is a measure of pressure both during the breath and also in between breaths. Because the breath is shorter, more time is spent at the lower pressure between breaths (PEEP level) and consequently the pressure overall tends to drop. Both flow and flow pattern refer to Volume Control breath styles only, as Pressure Control breath styles have no set flow rate or pattern.

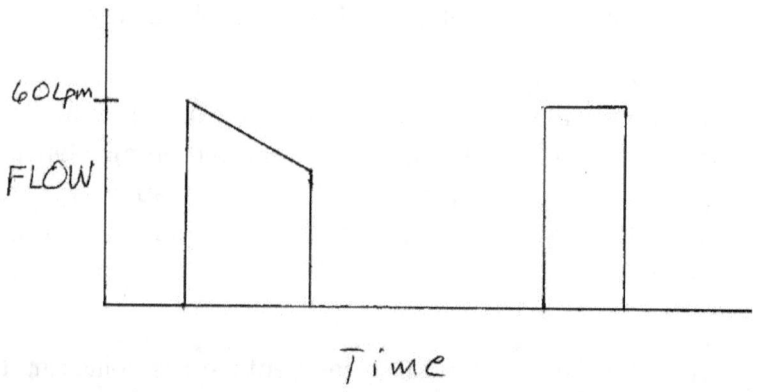

Fig 1. Decelerating Flow waveform on left and square waveform on right. Both are set at flow rates of 60 lpm and identical tidal volumes. Note the shortened duration of the breath when delivered with a square wave. Only the inspiratory portion of the waveform is depicted here.

Generally speaking, the decelerating waveform is more physiologic and comfortable for the patient, and hence it is what is used more often. There is usually not a very good reason to use the square wave, other than for taking measurements of airway resistance (Raw).

Trigger setting

For the ventilator to deliver an assisted breath, it needs to sense an inspiratory effort from the patient. This can be in the form of either a flow or pressure drop. Commonly, a flow of 2-3 lpm or a pressure drop of 2-3cm H20 is used. If a higher setting is used, this may increase work of breathing for the patient, as the patient will have to work more to generate the higher flow or pressure. Rarely, a higher setting is required due to the patient's heart beat or tremor causing autocycling of the ventilator. This may happen if the heart beat or tremor is dynamic enough to displace enough lung in order to cause a flow in the circuit.

Fraction of inspired oxygen (FiO2)

Percent of oxygen delivered.

Positive end expiratory pressure (PEEP)

Positive end expiratory pressure. Similar to CPAP when using noninvasive ventilation. This is the background pressure on top of which the ventilator delivers the breath.

I:E ratio or Inspiratory time (I-time)

In normal spontaneous breathing, the I:E ratio is 1:2 or 1:3. This represents the fact that normally one spends most of the time in exhalation, or at rest after exhalation. In AC mode, the ratio is not set by the user, but is a dependent variable determined by how the ventilator is set up. If a large tidal volume and a low flow rate are used, then the I:E ratio will increase, i.e., more time will be spent inspiring. If a low tidal volume and high flow rate are used, then the I:E ratio will decrease, and the patient will have more time to breathe out. In Pressure Control mode and VC+, the I-time is set by the user and is not a dependent variable.

3. Modes of Ventilation

The basic modes of ventilation one needs to be familiar with are: Assist Control-Volume Control (AC-VC), Assist Control-Pressure Control (AC-PC), Synchronized Intermittent Mechanical Ventilation (SIMV), Pressure Support (PS), and Volume Control plus (VC+)/Pressure Regulated Volume Control (PRVC). There are other modes of ventilation such as High Frequency Jet ventilation and Airway Pressure Release Ventilation (APRV) which are not commonly used, and so are not presented in this book. It should be noted that in common parlance, when someone says 'AC', they are referring to Assist Control-Volume Control.

To understand these different modes of ventilation, one needs to be familiar with the types of breaths the ventilator can deliver. CONCEPT: there are only *three* breath styles the ventilator can deliver: The Volume Control breath style, the Pressure Control breath style and the Pressure Support breath style. All the ventilator modes are comprised of one or more of these breath styles. Understanding these breath styles is key to getting a fundamental understanding of the different modes of ventilation, and to understanding exactly how the ventilator is delivering breaths to your patient.

The Volume Control breath style is where the ventilator delivers a set tidal volume. One sets the tidal volume, flow rate and flow waveform on the machine, and the ventilator delivers the breath according to those parameters. For example, one could set the Vt to 500, flow at 60 lpm, and waveform to decelerating. The peak and plateau pressures in this mode are *dependent* variables. That is, they will change if the patient's condition changes. If lung compliance worsens, then the ventilator will still deliver the tidal volume, however, the Ppeak and Pplat will go up. Also, if an albuterol nebulizer is administered and the airway resistance drops, the tidal volume will remain the same but the peak pressure will drop. The ventilator delivers the volume and ignores the peak pressure.

There is the concept of 'cycle' that needs to be understood. When we speak of cycling, we are referring to what determines when the ventilator stops delivering the breath. In VC mode it is obvious. Once the set Vt is delivered, the ventilator stops pushing air into the patient and allows the patient to exhale. Hence this mode is volume 'cycled'. In Pressure Control, the inspiratory time is set by the user. Once the inspiratory time is reached, the ventilator stops delivering the pressure and allows the patient to exhale. Thus, Pressure Control is time 'cycled'. Pressure Support is neither volume nor time cycled. The ventilator delivers the set pressure, until the flow rate that the patient is inhaling at drops to a specified value that can be set by the user. Commonly this is 25%. Once flow slows to this level, the ventilator stops delivering pressure and allows the patient to exhale. This makes sense, because as a patient nears the end of their breath, their inspiratory flow slows down. This mode is flow 'cycled'.

In the Pressure Control breath style, the inspiratory pressure and I-time are set by the user. It is the tidal volume and flow that are *dependent* variables here, as opposed to Ppeak and Pplat which are the dependent variables in Volume Control ventilation. The ventilator will deliver the set pressure constantly, and with an essentially unlimited flow, until the set I-time is reached. If the patient takes a fast, deep breath in, the servo in the ventilator will increase flow to maintain the set airway pressure. If there is a loss of lung compliance, the inspiratory pressure remains the same, but the tidal volume will drop. As mentioned earlier, this mode is time cycled inasmuch as the ventilator stops delivering a breath when the set I-time is reached.

The Pressure Support breath style is where the inspiratory pressure is set by the user. The tidal volume, inspiratory time, flow rate, and respiratory rate are all variable and are not set by the user. This mode of ventilation will allow for the most variation in ventilatory support for the patient. The patient may take one breath that is 1200cc and lasts 1.5 seconds, followed by two breaths that are 200cc and last half a second. Similar to the Pressure Control breath style, the ventilator can deliver essentially unlimited flow in order to maintain the set airway pressure. Generally speaking, this breath style is not used by itself as a means of ventilation, although with enough set pressure it could. It is mostly used as a component of SIMV and in spontaneous breathing trials. This breath style is flow cycled, in that when the inspiratory flow drops to a specified level as the patient approaches the end of inhalation, the ventilator stops delivering the set pressure and allows the patient to exhale.

Now that we understand the breath styles that the ventilator can deliver, we can better understand the modes of ventilation. Let us start with understanding what Assist Control means.

Assist Control or AC is the basic algorithm the ventilator uses to deliver breaths. It is a combination of *control* breaths and *assisted* breaths. CONCEPT: with the exception of Pressure Support, all the common ventilator modes are run with this basic assist-control algorithm. This includes AC-VC, AC-PC, SIMV, and VC+/PRVC. It is the *breath styles* employed that create the different modes, not the underlying algorithm. Under the assist control algorithm, if one sets a respiratory rate of 12/min for example, the ventilator will deliver 1 breath every 5 seconds (60 seconds/12 = 5 seconds). These breaths are termed *Control* breaths because no patient effort is involved in triggering the breath. They are simply delivered in 5 second intervals. If no patient effort is sensed after 5 seconds, the ventilator will deliver the next breath. If the patient starts to inhale prior to the 5 second interval, the ventilator will detect the flow and deliver a breath. These breaths are termed *Assisted* breaths because the ventilator is *assisting* the patient effort by delivering a breath. Each mode is defined by what breath style is used for the control breath, and what breath style is used for the assisted breath.

AC-VC

AC-VC is the Volume Controlled breath style delivered under the AC setting. Both the control and the assisted breath are VC breath styles. If one sets the rate at 12 and Vt at 500, for example, the ventilator will deliver a 500cc Vt every 5 seconds. If the patient inspires before the 5 second mark, the ventilator will deliver the full, assisted 500cc tidal volume. A patient who is on neuromuscular blockade will receive exactly twelve 500cc breaths every minute. A patient who is anxious on the ventilator may receive many more than twelve 500cc breaths per minute, comprised of some assisted and some controlled breaths. Regardless of whether the breath is assisted or controlled, the tidal volume delivered is 500cc. See Fig 2.

SIMV

Synchronized Intermittent Mechanical Ventilation (SIMV) is a mode of ventilation utilizing the Volume Control and Pressure Support breath styles. A better name for this mode would have been AC-VC/PS because that is exactly what it is. It can also be used with the Pressure Control breath style instead of the VC breath style, but this is not commonly done. It is not normally used in the MICU, but one should be familiar with it, as it is sometimes used by the anesthesia and surgical services, and occasionally someone will arrive out of the OR on SIMV.

SIMV uses the Volume Control breath style for the control breath and the Pressure Support breath style for the assisted breath. If the respiratory rate is set at 12, then it will deliver the VC style breath every 5 seconds. The difference between this mode and AC-VC, is what happens when the patient triggers a breath. In

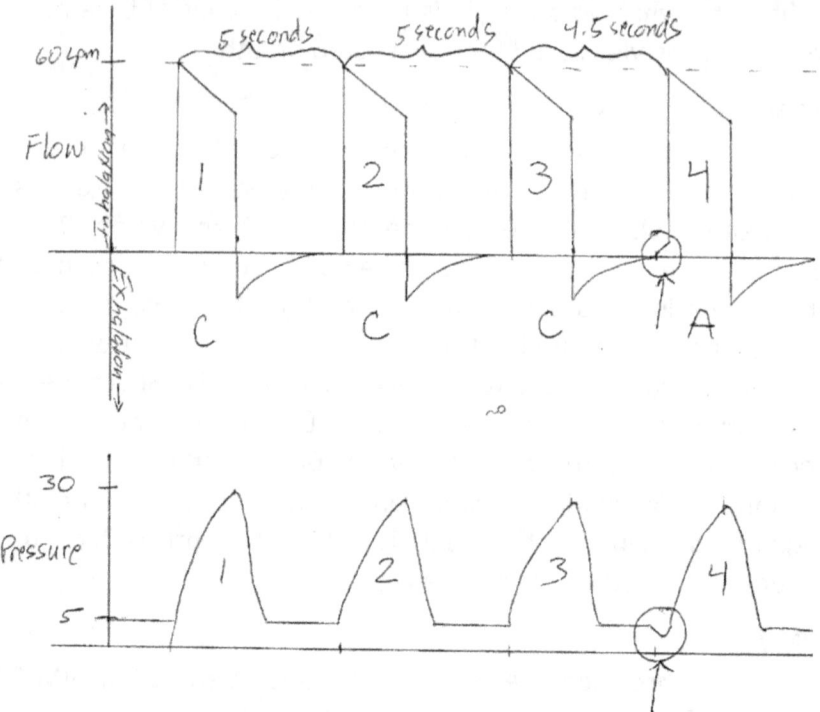

Fig 2. Flow and pressure waveforms for a patient on AC-VC rate=12, VT=500, Peep=5, decelerating flow set at 60 lpm. Breaths 1,2 and 3 are controlled breaths. Breath 4 occurs a little earlier and is an assisted breath. Note the circled area in the top portion denoting the flow generated by the patient to trigger breath 4. The circled portion in the bottom part of the figure shows the pressure dip caused by the patient triggering a breath.

AC-VC mode, the ventilator will deliver the assisted breath using a VC breath style. In SIMV, the patient triggered breaths are delivered in the Pressure Support breath style. The user sets the VC breath style tidal volume and the Pressure Support breath style set pressure. Commonly, the Pressure Support is set at 10cm H20. As the patient triggered breaths are delivered as Pressure Support, there is less offloading of the patient's work of breathing in SIMV

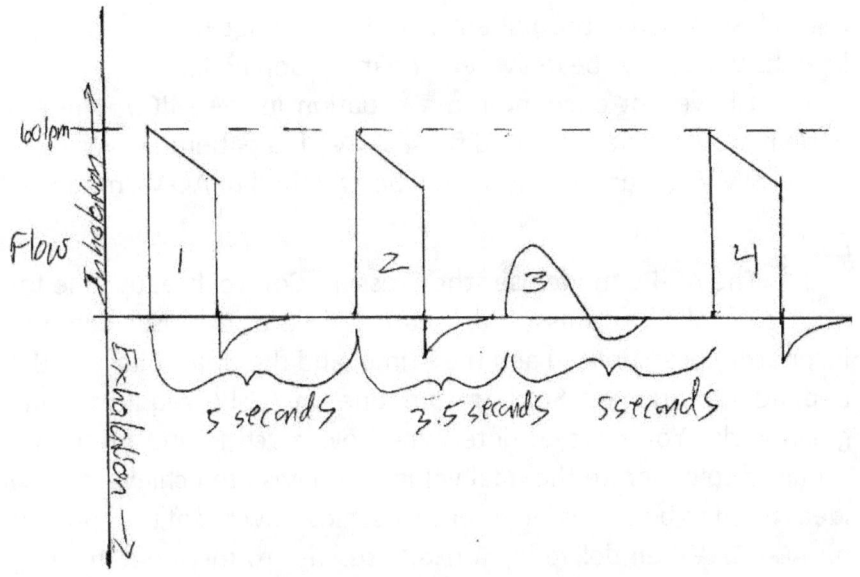

Figure 3. This is a patient on SIMV set at RR=12, flow at 60 lpm, decelerating waveform and PS=10. Breaths 1,2 and 4 are VC style breaths. Breath 3 is a patient triggered breath and hence is a PS style breath. Note the smaller overall flow and hence volume in breath 3. Compare breath 3 in this figure to breath 4 in Fig 2. Both are assisted breaths.

as compared to AC-VC. If the patient is on neuromuscular blockade and not triggering any breaths, SIMV and AC-VC will perform identically (Fig 3). It should be noted that although SIMV utilizes the Assist/Control algorithm, it is modified to ensure that the set rate of VC breaths is always delivered. If the patient is under neuromuscular blockade on SIMV set at a rate of 10, for example, the ventilator will deliver exactly 10 controlled VC style breaths. If the patient is breathing spontaneously at a rate of 40 on SIMV set at a rate of 10, the ventilator will deliver 10 breaths as assisted VC style breaths and 30 breaths as assisted PS style breaths. On SIMV, regardless of what the patient is doing, the set rate of VC style breaths will always be delivered - no more and no less.

I have not encountered a situation in the MICU where a patient would have benefited from SIMV. If a patient arrives from OR on SIMV, generally they should be switched to AC-VC mode.

AC-PC

The AC-PC mode uses the Pressure Control breath style for both controlled and assisted breaths. Here, the user sets the inspiratory pressure (Pi) and the I-time, and the tidal volume is the dependent variable. Starting someone on AC-PC requires some guesswork. You have to determine how much Pi and I-time are required to generate the tidal volume you wish to achieve. A few ideas need to be discussed prior to learning how to set up a patient on AC-PC. When delivering a fixed pressure to the lung, the lung will inflate to a point where the elastic recoil of the lung balances the inflation pressure. When the lung reaches this point, prolonging the insufflation time further will not increase the Vt. This essentially becomes a breath-hold maneuver or end inspiratory pause beyond this point of maximal inflation. Also, it should be noted that the shorter the I-time is set at, the higher the Pi that will be needed to insufflate the lung to goal Vt. The air needs to be pushed in faster to get to the goal Vt in the shorter timeframe. Keeping these ideas in mind, let us discuss how to set a patient up on AC-PC.

I would suggest starting with a Pi of 20cm H2O and an I-time of 0.85 seconds. Most of the time, this will get you close to where you need to be. Titrate the Pi to get to the goal Vt. If the measured Vt is too low, then increase the pressure. If it is too high, then decrease it. Once goal Vt is reached, one of three scenarios will be present:

    a) Goal Vt is achieved prior to I-time being reached. There will be a time of zero flow at the end of the breath. If

this is the case, then decrease I-time until the breath ends when the I-time expires (Fig 4).
b) Goal Vt is achieved with Pi > 30cm H2O and no I-time at zero flow present. Here, an excessive Pi is required to achieve goal Vt. If this occurs, I suggest increasing I-time in 0.05 second increments. If Vt goes up, then decrease Pi as able, until you can hopefully get Pi to < 30. Increase I-time until further increases in Vt cease to occur. In the stiff lung, it may not be possible to get to a Pi of <30, but one should try to get to goal Vt with as little pressure as possible. If zero flow at the end of the breath develops, then you know further increases in I-time will not increase Vt.
c) Goal Vt is achieved with Pi < 30cm H20 and no time at zero flow present. Here we are at goal, and no further adjustment needs to be made

The cutoff of 30cm H2O here is arbitrary, but generally I try to keep Pi less than this if possible. Remember, we always try to ventilate the patient with as little pressure, volume, and oxygen as we are able to.

The main advantage of Pressure Control, is that in some patients with a very stiff lung or unstable respiratory pattern, it can improve synchrony. This is in part because the servo can deliver unlimited and variable flow rates, as opposed to the fixed rates of AC-VC. If you are having trouble with ventilator synchrony on AC-VC, it is worthwhile to try AC-PC and see if the patient looks more comfortable on it.

VC+/PRVC

VC+, also called PRVC on some machines, is a mode which uses the Pressure Control breath style for both the controlled and assisted breaths. A better name would have been AC-PC+ because that is exactly what it is. It is a modified version of AC-PC. It is a time cycled, unlimited flow breath. This mode is best described as 'auto-titrating' Pressure Control. The respiratory rate and I-time are set by the user, but instead of setting the inspiratory pressure (Pi), one sets the desired tidal volume. The ventilator then titrates the Pi automatically to achieve the desired Vt. In most cases this mode replaces AC-PC, in that it functions similarly to AC-PC, but it has the benefit of generating a more stable Vt in the face of changing lung compliance or airway resistance. I preferentially use

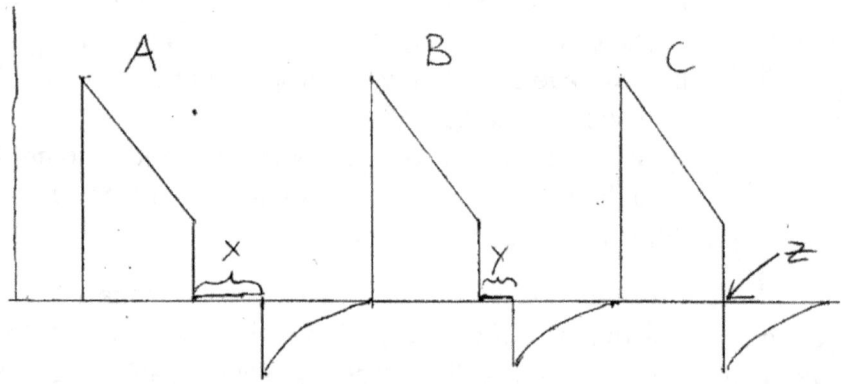

Fig. 4. Decreasing the I-time until the Vt is delivered in synchrony with the I-time. 'A' represents an I-time of 1 second. Notice zero flow at 'x'. 'B' represents an I-time of 0.9 seconds. Notice zero flow at 'y'. 'C' represents an I-time of 0.85 seconds. Notice no time at zero flow- 'just right'.

VC+ over AC-PC in cases where the Pressure Control breath style produces better ventilator synchrony.

Pressure Support (PS)
    PS isn't commonly used as a means to ventilate a patient. It could be used that way if one sets the pressure high enough. It has no controlled breaths-all breaths in this mode are assisted breaths. It is generally used as a component of SIMV, as discussed earlier,

and as the support method during a spontaneous breathing trial, which we will discuss in a later chapter.

The following chart summarizes the breath styles employed by the different ventilator modes:

Mode	Control breath	Assisted breath
AC-VC	VC	VC
AC-PC	PC	PC
SIMV	VC	PS/VC
VC+/PRVC	PC	PC
PS	None	PS

4. Respiratory Mechanics and Concepts

Compliance

Lung compliance refers to the ease of inflation of the lung. A compliant lung will inflate easily, with only a minimal amount of pressure. A noncompliant or 'stiff' lung as seen in ARDS, will only inflate a little with the same amount of pressure. Many lung ailments such as ARDS, pneumonia, or pulmonary edema will worsen or decrease lung compliance.

The formula for lung compliance is as follows:

$$C = \text{Change in Volume}/\text{Change in Pressure}$$

For patients on a ventilator, it is practically expressed as:

$$C = \text{Tidal Volume}/(\text{Plateau Pressure - PEEP})$$

The plateau pressure - PEEP is also known as 'Driving Pressure' so:

$$C = \text{Tidal Volume}/\text{Driving Pressure}$$

In the ICU, it is not possible to tease out lung compliance from the total system compliance, so what we are really measuring is respiratory system compliance. A normal respiratory system compliance is 50-100cc/cm H20. This means that for every cm H20 pressure applied to the system, the lung should inflate by 50-100 cc.

Airway Resistance (Raw)

The resistance to flow in the airway is calculated by the following equation:

$$Raw = (Ppeak - Pplat)/\text{Flow L/sec}$$

The measurement needs to be done with a square wave flow pattern with a Volume Control breath style. Generally speaking, < 10cm H2O/L/sec is considered normal for a healthy person on a ventilator. Conditions that can increase Raw include asthma, COPD, bronchospasm, and pneumonia with significant secretions. A shortcut to this calculation is to set the flow at 60 lpm with a square wave. On this setting, the Raw simply equates to Ppeak - Pplat, as 60 lpm is 1 L/second, so the denominator of the equation becomes 1.

Positive End Expiratory Pressure (PEEP)

PEEP is the background airway circuit pressure on top of which the ventilator delivers a breath. The pressure in the circuit will not drop below this level, other than for short spurts of time when the servo in the ventilator is trying to catch up with pressure fluctuations. Commonly it is set at 5-20cm H20. Its purpose is to help recruit alveoli, decrease atelectasis, and hence help improve oxygenation (Fig 5).

PEEP and FiO2 are the main determinants of oxygenation. Usually PEEP is set to 'physiologic PEEP' of 5cm H20. This 'physiologic' setting was based on the notion that in a spontaneously breathing normal patient, the natural flow limitation of the partially closed glottis produced a small amount of PEEP. However, at the end of a normal relaxed breath in a normal person, there is minimal to no flow, making this concept suspect, as if there is no flow with an open glottis there cannot be any PEEP. Mainly, it is just historical precedent that explains why the PEEP is usually initially set at 5cm H20. Generally speaking, the higher the FiO2 required, the higher the PEEP should be set at.

A reasonable PEEP table would be:

FiO2	PEEP
40%	5
50%	8
60%	10
70%	12
80%	14
>80%	14-20

There is not very much science to this. Some studies[1] have shown similar outcomes in ARDS regardless of whether high or low PEEP was used. In my practice, I use a PEEP level approximating what is in the above table. Maximum alveolar recruitment sometimes takes several hours, but de-recruitment can happen quite quickly, so when weaning down PEEP it should generally be done slowly.

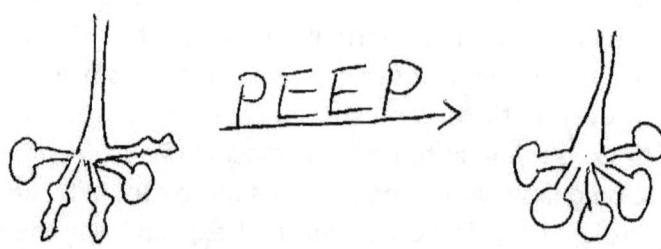

Fig 5. Collapsed alveoli on left and recruited alveoli on right after the application of PEEP. Notice how PEEP 'pops open' the alveoli thereby improving oxygenation.

PEEP also has hemodynamic effects. It can decrease preload by increasing intrathoracic pressure, and thereby decreasing venous return. It also decreases afterload by decreasing transmural pressure across the left ventricle. This has a combined effect similar to giving someone nitrates + an ace-inhibitor. It will tend to decrease blood pressure some. It also tends to improve pulmonary edema. If PEEP is high enough, in some patients, it can impair RV function by increasing pulmonary vascular resistance[2], but this is not commonly encountered clinically.

Autopeep

Dynamic Hyperinflation is a pathologic process which occurs when a patient isn't able to exhale fully prior to taking the next breath. The result of this process is autopeep. Autopeep, in a way, represents air being trapped in the lung. It tends to occur in patients with airway obstruction, such as COPD and asthma, where airflow during expiration is impaired and much slower, and hence the patient doesn't have enough time to expire to FRC prior to the ventilator giving the next breath. It may also occur in the normal lung if respiratory rate is set very high. In many patients in the ICU on a ventilator with a RR >30, there is likely to be some degree of autopeep.

Deleterious Effects of Autopeep

Autopeep can cause harm in a number of ways. It can increase airway pressures, and therefore increase the likelihood of barotrauma. It can increase Pplat by hyperinflating the lung to a stiffer point on the compliance curve. It can cause hypotension by increasing intrathoracic pressure and decreasing venous return. It can also increase work of breathing. For a patient to trigger a breath on a ventilator, they must generate a flow in the circuit that the ventilator can detect. Autopeep causes a flow out of the lung at the end of the breath-an expiratory flow. The ventilator needs to sense an inspiratory flow in order to release an assisted breath.

If the autopeep trapped in the patient's alveoli and small airways is, for example, 5cm H20, then the patient's diaphragm and chest muscles will need to contract hard enough in the beginning of inspiration to overcome that 5cm H20 pressure, before the pressure in the main airways drops below the ventilator circuit pressure to cause a flow into the patient's lung that the ventilator can detect. That extra effort adds to the patient's work of breathing. It makes it harder for the patient to trigger a breath on the ventilator.

Recognizing Autopeep

There are a few ways to detect autopeep on the ventilator. If you press the end-expiratory pause button, the ventilator will delay the next breath, and instead wait and measure the pressure that builds up in the circuit as the air trapped as autopeep slowly drains out of the lung. It will then output that number in cm H20 pressure. This measurement is problematic, however, as the ventilator needs time to take this measurement. Unless the patient is breathing very slowly, or on neuromuscular blockade, this maneuver may not work. Displayed graphically on the ventilator, an end-expiratory pause maneuver would look like fig 6.

Another way to gauge autopeep is to look at the flow waveform. The flow should return to zero at the end of a breath. If it doesn't, then autopeep is present (Fig 7). No special maneuver is required here, only observation of the flow graphic. The higher the expiratory flow is just prior to onset of the next breath, the more autopeep is present. Sometimes it is helpful to magnify the flow graphic in order to see this more clearly.

You can also detect autopeep by looking at how the patient is interacting with the ventilator. If the patient is autopeeping significantly, there will be a delay between when the patient starts to inhale and when the breath is delivered by the ventilator. This delay is the time it takes for the respiratory musculature to generate enough negative pressure in the chest, to overcome the

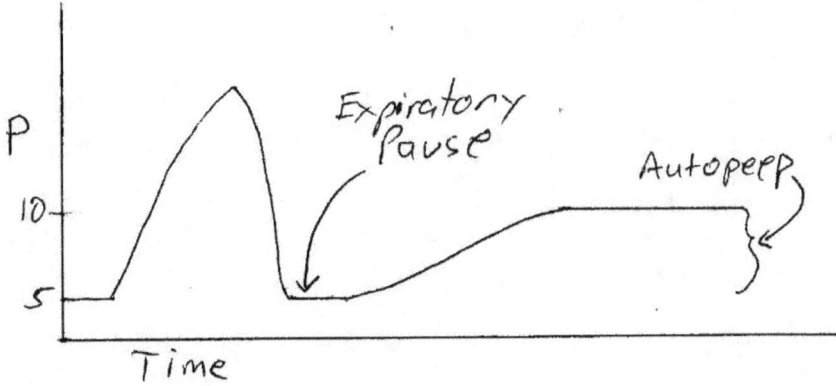

Fig 6. End-expiratory pause maneuver occurs at arrow. Autopeep measured here is 5cm H2O above PEEP.

autopeep present in the lung, to create a flow into the lung that the ventilator will detect. In severe cases, the patient can attempt to take in a breath but fail, due to the level of autopeep surpassing the intrathoracic pressure drop produced by the inspiratory effort. Here the patient is 'locked out' of the breath and doesn't trigger the breath at all. In some cases, the patient is 'locked out' of every other breath. This condition was termed 'respiratory flutter with a 2:1 block' by one of my old (and very wise) pulmonology attendings.

After detecting the presence of autopeep in a patient, one needs to decide what to do about it. Treating bronchospasm and airway obstruction with steroids and nebulizers is prudent. If this fails to improve things, then other maneuvers can be done. Firstly, one needs to determine if the autopeep is problematic. If Ppeak is <30, blood pressure is ok, and the patient is not having ventilator synchrony issues, then nothing really needs to be done. If autopeep is causing negative consequences, then some action is warranted.

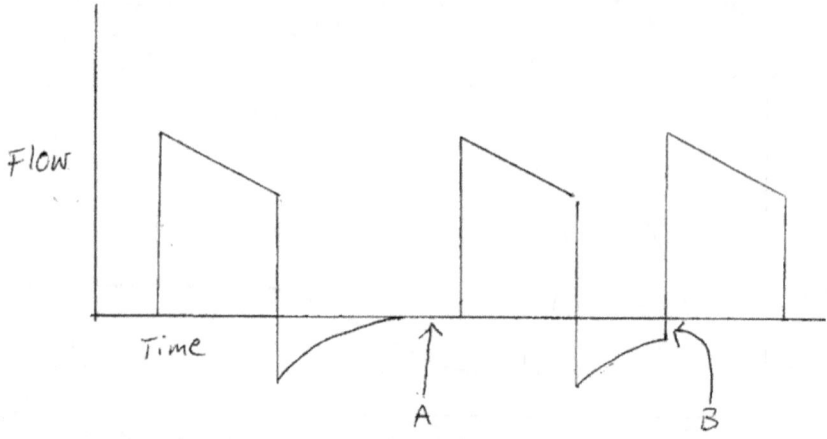

Fig 7. Autopeep visualized on a flow graphic. At 'A' there is no flow prior to the next breath. This is normal. At 'B' there is flow present. This represents dynamic hyperinflation/autopeep.

The cornerstone of managing autopeep lies in increasing the time the patient has to expire. By far, the best way to do this is to decrease the respiratory rate. If the patient is initiating breaths, then sedation can help to decrease the patient-initiated breaths. The second most helpful maneuver is to decrease the tidal volume. Other measures such as increasing flow rate and changing to a square wave are less helpful.

'Canceling' autopeep with extrinsic PEEP can be tried. This can decrease the work-of-breathing problem associated with autopeep, but will not actually decrease the amount of autopeep present, and hence will not help with airway pressure issues or hypotension issues. What one attempts to do is increase PEEP from the ventilator so that it matches the amount of autopeep in the patient. If the pressure in the trapped air in the lung and the pressure in the circuit are equal, then it takes little effort to generate enough inspiratory flow to trigger a breath. This is more of an interesting physiologic point and less of a clinically effective maneuver, as its overall impact in improving the patient's situation is modest.

As a side note, when patients with severe COPD perform pursed lipped breathing, they are in part splinting open their airways to improve exhalation, and in part canceling autopeep with extrinsic PEEP to help with inspiratory work of breathing.

Dead Space

Total dead space in the lung is comprised of anatomic dead space and physiologic dead space. Anatomic dead space is essentially all of the respiratory tract from the nose on down that does not have alveoli. Physiologic dead space refers to parts of the lung with alveoli that do not participate in gas exchange due to a lack of blood flow. This occurs in West zone 1 of the lung, where pressure in the alveolus is higher than the pulmonary capillary pressure, and hence no blood flow occurs there. There is ventilation but no perfusion, and hence no gas can be exchanged. It also occurs in many disease states such as COPD, pneumonia, and pulmonary embolus, that cause a mismatch between blood flow and ventilation to alveoli.

On a ventilator circuit, the dead space starts at the 'Y' fitting. This is where fresh air and exhaled air are exchanged, and is the anatomic equivalent of your nose. (Fig 8).

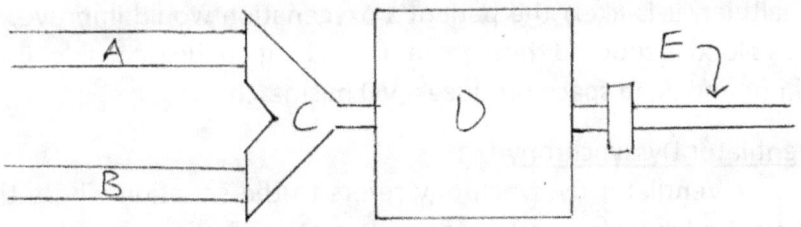

Fig 8. 'A' is the inspiratory limb of ventilator tubing. 'B' is the expiratory limb of ventilator tubing. 'C' is the Y adapter where dead space begins. 'D' is the heat and moisture exchanger. 'E' is the endotracheal tube.

Generally speaking, an increase in dead space will cause an increase in PCO2. The prototype state for dead space is a pulmonary embolism. When a PE is present, there is no blood flow to the affected area, but ventilation to that area continues. In the case of a PE, hypercapnia is rare, as most people hyperventilate some due to the PE. Also, due to atelectasis and hemorrhage, hypoxemia is usually present.

Shunt

Shunt is, in a way, the opposite of dead space. It is where there is blood flow not exposed to functional alveoli. Think of a patent foramen ovale (PFO). Blood flows right past the lung and picks up no oxygen. Consolidation and atelectasis also produce a shunt, as blood flows past alveoli that aren't filled with air. The effect of shunt is hypoxemia. Generally speaking, if a shunt is present, likely there is some increase in dead space as well, and vice versa. One should keep in mind that blood flow to the lung is affected by gravity. There is more blood flow in gravitationally dependent portions of the lung. If a patient has a severe right-sided pneumonia with consolidation of much of the lung, one would have significant shunt present. If the physician places pillows under the shoulder and hip of the right side of the patient, this would cause the left lung to be more gravitationally dependent, and more blood flow would pass through the left lung. If the left lung was relatively healthier, it is likely the patient's oxygenation would improve, as less blood is shunted through damaged lung on the right side. Both shunt and dead space produce a VQ mismatch.

Ventilator Dyssynchrony

Ventilator dyssynchrony refers to the situation where the patient's breathing pattern doesn't match what the ventilator is providing. Potential consequences of poor synchrony include self-inflicted lung injury, derecruitment, and barotrauma. Here we will list some common causes of dyssynchrony.

A) Inadequate sedation

If a patient is agitated, sometimes they will try to expire prior to the ventilator completing the breath. This generally sets off the peak pressure alarm. This problem is usually fairly obvious at the bedside. The solution is to sedate the patient better.

B) Breath stacking

Breath stacking refers to a patient inhaling two separate ventilator generated tidal volumes on a single breath. As a result, the true Vt is twice the set Vt (Fig 9). The reason this occurs is the patient's native requirement for Vt is not being met by the ventilator. One way to fix this is to increase the set Vt. For example, if you have an ARDS patient you are trying to perform low Vt ventilation on, and calculated they needed a Vt of 360cc but they are breath stacking, then the true Vt is 720cc. Increasing Vt to 400cc may alleviate the problem. Being 20-40cc above goal is far better than delivering twice the goal Vt. Sedating the patient may also improve this, as sedation will decrease the respiratory drive. Decreasing the flow rate may help as well. This allows the patient more time to inspire, and in some cases can resolve the issue.

C) Autopeep

Autopeep can cause dyssynchrony. Please see earlier discussion of autopeep.

D) Autocycling of the ventilator

Autocycling refers to the ventilator delivering an assisted breath without the patient actually triggering the ventilator. It is a false trigger of the ventilator. If the flow trigger is set low, then the patient's heart beat and the flow that is generated by the heart's compression and expansion of adjacent lung can trigger the ventilator in some patients. The solution here is to increase the triggering flow or pressure. If enough condensation builds up in

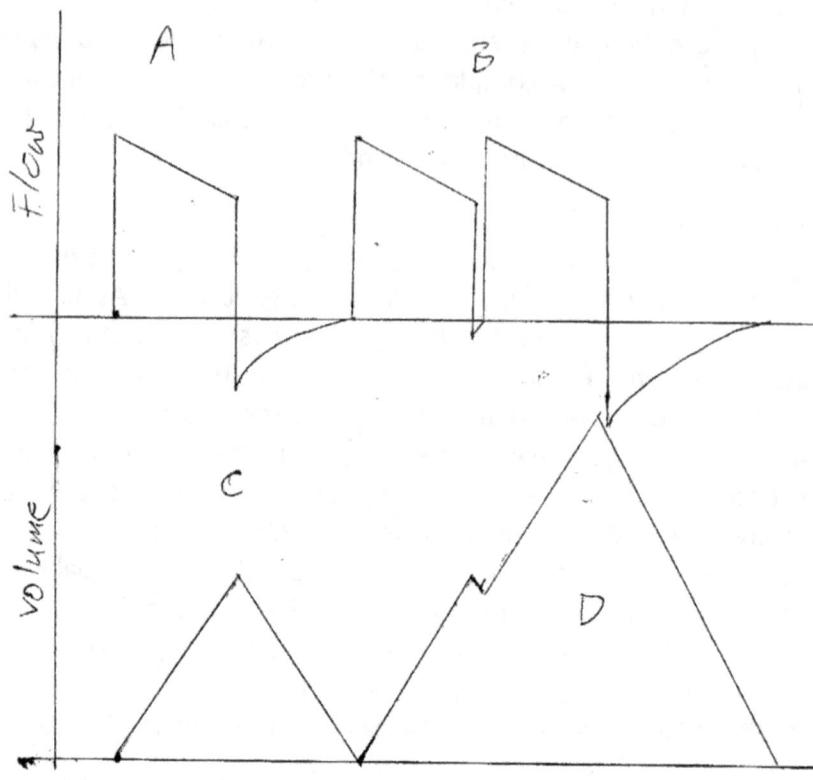

Fig 9. Breath stacking. 'A' is a normal breath flow waveform. 'B' is a breath stacked breath flow waveform. 'C' is a normal Vt. 'D' is a breath stacked Vt.

the ventilator tubing, it can slosh around and generate a flow that can trigger the ventilator- the so called 'water hammer' effect. Disconnecting the tubing and draining the accumulated water solves the problem. A pneumothorax with a large air leak managed with a chest tube to suction can cause autocycling if the suction applied through the chest tube pulls enough air through the leak to trigger the ventilator.

E) Insufficient flow/ Flow starvation

Some patients require a very high flow rate and may outstrip the set flow on the ventilator. This will be noticeable as a paradoxical breathing effort similar to what it would look like if someone tried to inhale against a closed glottis. The vent pressure tracing will show a dip in pressure during the breath (Fig 10). Normally, the airway pressure rises until the breath is finished. This problem can be remedied by increasing the set flow rate on AC-VC mode. Also, changing to AC-PC or VC+ will alleviate the problem, as these modes automatically adjust flow to suit the patient's needs.

Plateau Pressure (Pplat)

Plateau pressure is a measure of the force of the lung's elastic recoil when insufflated with the set tidal volume. It is measured when there is no flow in the system, which excludes any pressure component related to Raw. To measure Pplat, one does an inspiratory hold maneuver (Fig 11). This is performed by pressing the inspiratory hold button on the ventilator. The ventilator waits until the completed Vt is delivered, and then holds the breath in the patient while measuring the pressure in the circuit. The ARDSnet study identified a Pplat <30 as a safe pressure. Increases in Vt and decreases in lung compliance are things that will increase Pplat.

Driving Pressure (Dp)

Driving pressure is the difference between the plateau pressure and the PEEP (Dp = Pplat - PEEP). Generally speaking, in the lung-injured patient, a Dp <20 is a reasonable goal[3]. This metric is useful for patients on high levels of PEEP, as it is difficult to obtain a Pplat of <30 if the patient is on a PEEP of 20. If the Pplat is >30 but the Dp <20 you are probably OK. The reality is that these sharp cutoffs are somewhat artificial. The less distension and pressure you can use and still accomplish the goal, the better. In a way, the Dp is a good fallback parameter in patients where you can't achieve a Pplat of <30 by adjusting the Vt.

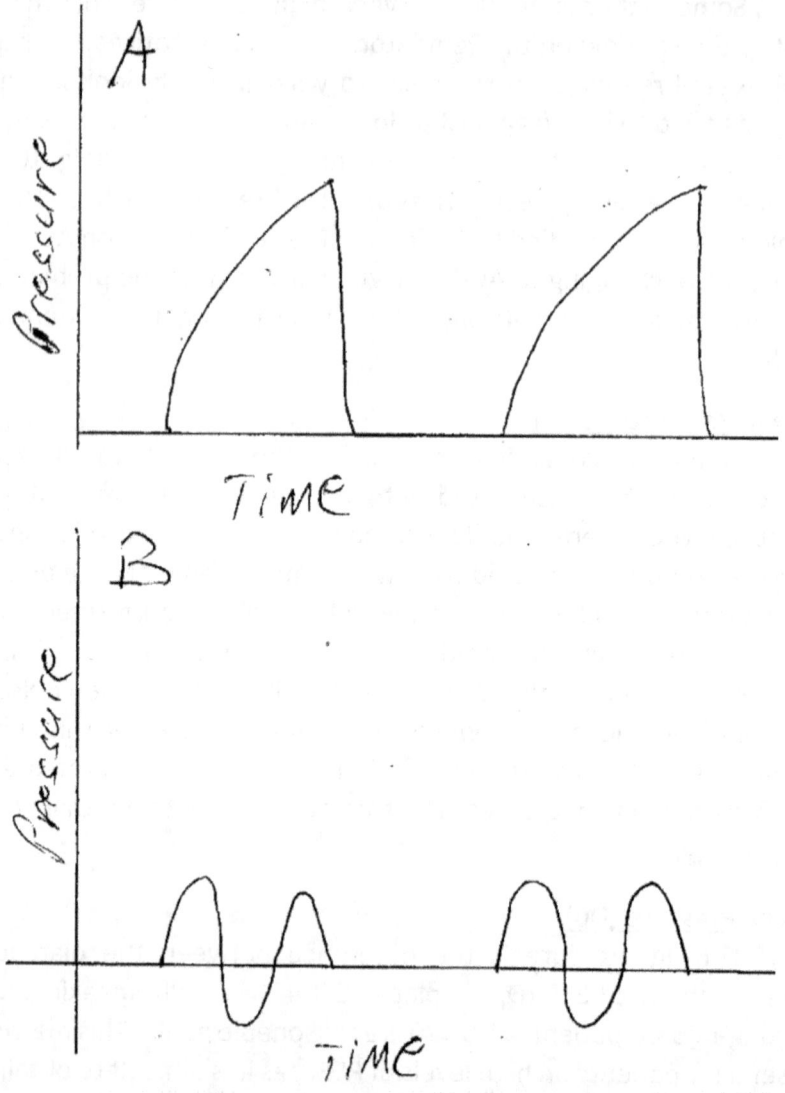

Fig 10. Pressure v time curves in normal breath 'A' and insufficient flow breath 'B'. Note the pressure dip in panel B.

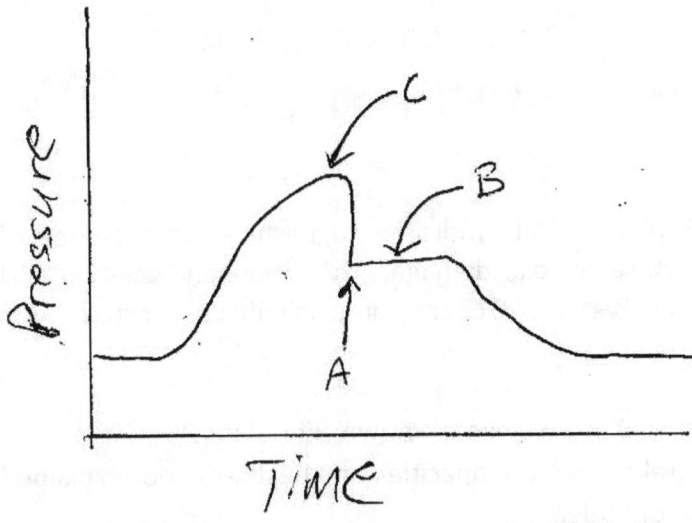

Fig 11. Plateau pressure measured after an inspiratory hold maneuver. 'A' is the point the inspiratory hold starts. 'B' is the plateau pressure. 'C' is the peak airway pressure for the breath.

Permissive Hypercapnia

The term permissive hypercapnia refers to a ventilator strategy which allows for elevated PCO2 levels, in order to achieve more important ventilator parameter endpoints such as low Vt and Pplat. It is founded in the understanding that high PCO2 levels and moderate levels of acidosis are well tolerated by the body, and therefore do not justify increases in Vt or Pplat in order to correct them. As long as the pH >/= 7.2, the minute ventilation does not need to be adjusted further. This concept is important in disease states such as ARDS and status asthmaticus, where many times, trying to drive the lung to produce a normal pH and PCO2 would likely cause significant harm.

5. Ventilation in Specific Circumstances

ARDS

ARDS is a clinical syndrome suggesting the presence of underlying diffuse alveolar damage. The European Society of ICU Medicine met in Berlin in 2012 and came up with consensus criteria for ARDS as follows[4]:

1. Onset within 1 week of a known clinical insult
2. Bilateral pulmonary opacities on chest x-ray not explained by chf or atelectasis
3. Exclusion of chf
4. Moderate to severe impairment of oxygenation in the presence of at least 5 of PEEP

    Mild: *P/F ratio <300, but >200

    Moderate: P/F ratio <200, but >100

    Severe: P/F ratio <100

    *P/F ratio is ratio of PO2/FiO2

The underlying strategies in ARDS are largely determined by the ARDSnet studies[5]. The main goals are a Vt of 6cc/kg ideal body weight and a Pplat of <30cm H20. This is known as lung protective ventilation. Sacrifices one makes here in terms of PCO2, and consequently pH, are termed permissive hypercapnia. One starts by setting the Vt to 6cc/kg. This is the first goal. One then sees what the Pplat is. If the Pplat is <30, then one is at goal. If the Pplat is >30cm H20, then the Vt is dropped further to reach the Pplat goal. As the Vt is decreased to try to achieve the Pplat goal, invariably the PCO2 starts to climb and the pH starts to drop. One can ignore the PCO2, but if the pH drops to less than 7.2, one can increase the RR to increase Ve and decrease PCO2. If RR is maximized (usually in the low 30's-because, as discussed, once it is raised higher than this then autopeep many times starts to develop) and the Pplat goal is not able to be reached without dropping pH to <7.2, then one can look at the driving pressure. If Driving pressure is <20, then one can say the goal has been achieved. If both Pplat and driving pressure are not at goal, and pH has become a problem, then one can either try to increase RR further, at the risk of causing autopeep, or one can administer bicarbonate. Also, one can leave it alone, as a reasonable effort has been attempted to reach the lung protective goals.

Titrate FiO2 and PEEP to keep O2 sat >/= 90%. There is no benefit in hyperoxygenating patients. Please see the PEEP table described in the previous chapter.

Status Asthmaticus

Status asthmaticus refers to severe and refractory bronchoconstriction in a patient with asthma. Probably one of the most difficult to manage patients from a ventilator standpoint is the severe asthmatic. The difficulty is that sometimes the autopeep and airway resistance are so severe that a reasonable amount of ventilation is hard to achieve without creating very high Ppeak and Pplat. The strategy here is to maximize the time the patient has to expire, in order to minimize the deleterious effects of dynamic hyperinflation. One should try to decrease RR as much as possible. Heavy sedation and/or NM blockade is sometimes necessary as the respiratory acidosis will cause the patient to try to initiate breaths. The next best thing to adjust is the Vt, in terms of increasing expiratory time. A lower Vt can be exhaled faster. Adjusting flow waveform and flow rate may have some beneficial effects but it is the RR that will contribute most.

Here again, a pH of >7.2 is acceptable. Consider using propofol or ketamine as a sedative, as these drugs have some bronchodilator effects. Anecdotally, in refractory cases, calling anesthesia and having them hook the patient up to the anesthesia machine and administering an inhaled anesthetic for a few hours may help, as the inhaled anesthetic has a bronchodilator effect.

<u>Increased ICP</u>

Here the strategy is to minimize increases in ICP due to the patient being on the ventilator and receiving positive pressure. Positive pressure ventilation increases ICP by: 1) increasing thoracic pressure and decreasing cerebral venous outflow 2) decreasing CSF outflow and 3) by decreasing MAP and causing cerebral vasodilation. It is instructive to watch what happens to ICP when PEEP is changed on a patient who has an ICP monitor in place. As PEEP is increased, the ICP climbs in real time. Many times, it is recommended to ventilate with a PEEP of zero to minimize this. Good sedation to minimize ventilator dyssynchrony and coughing is important.

One generally should aim for a normal PCO_2 and pH here. Hyperventilation to a PCO_2 of around thirty can be tried, as this will decrease ICP by causing cerebral vasoconstriction. However, this maneuver will also decrease cerebral blood flow, potentially injuring threatened areas of the brain. This should only be done to buy time in a patient with impending herniation who is on their way to the OR.

6. Liberation from Mechanical Ventilation

'Liberation' has replaced the term 'weaning' when speaking of discontinuing mechanical ventilation on a patient. This is because there really isn't any weaning done. The patient is either ready to come off the ventilator, or is not. When contemplating liberating someone from the ventilator, one first needs to clinically assess if the patient is ready to be taken off the ventilator. The following conditions need to be met:

1. Reverse a reversible process. Did we fix whatever landed the patient on the ventilator in the first place? Did the pneumonia get better? Did bronchoconstriction improve? This process is a combination of bedside evaluation and knowing the natural history of the disease. If you just intubated someone with IPF, don't expect to get him off the ventilator the next day.
2. Hemodynamically stable. Generally speaking, the patient should be off of pressors. Although being on low-dose pressors that are getting weaned off is also acceptable. Mostly this applies to patients in septic shock, as being in shock is likely part of the reason the patient got intubated in the first place. Many post-CABG patients get taken off the ventilator while still on pressors, as the shock is due to cardiac depression in isolation, and not a manifestation of a systemic/global disorder.
3. Metabolically stable. The patient should not be significantly acidotic. One of the benefits of mechanical ventilation is the ability to better control the patient's acid-base balance.
4. Able to protect the airway. This boils down to three parameters:
    a) Awake and alert and able to follow commands.
    b) Manageable secretions-either oral or endotracheal. An older patient will not be able to manage secretions as well

as a younger, stronger patient. Accumulation of secretions in the upper airway will lead to aspiration and/or atelectasis, and possible reintubation. If you are suctioning the patient hourly, then the patient is likely not ready to be extubated.
- c) Core muscle strength. This is often overlooked or ignored. Patients can be wide awake but have minimal core muscle strength. Just because the patient's brain is ok does not mean that they can breathe well. Without good strength, patients can't cough well or clear secretions, and will be prone to atelectasis or aspiration. A good way to test this is to ask the patient to lift their head off the bed. If the patient can do this, then chances are the strength needed is there.

5. Minimal ventilator settings.
   - a) FiO2 of 40%
   - b) PEEP of 5
   - c) Minute ventilation of <15 and RR <30

Once these parameters are met, the patient can proceed to a spontaneous breathing trial. CONCEPT: A spontaneous breathing trial is a SIMULATION of a patient breathing without an endotracheal tube and without a ventilator. It is important to conceptualize it as a simulation. There are two common ways to run the simulation.

1. <u>T-Piece</u>

A T-Piece is a T-shaped plastic connector one can attach to the end of an endotracheal tube. Oxygen is delivered through tubing that looks similar to ventilator tubing. The patient breathes in from the continuous flow of air/O2 mixture that passes through the T-Piece. See Fig 12.

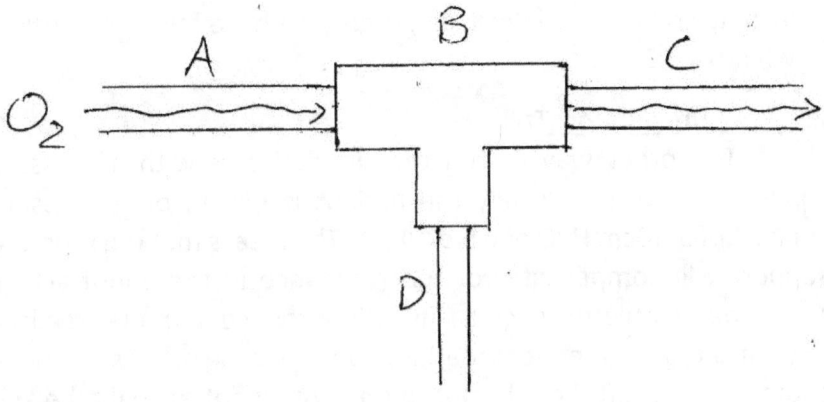

Fig 12. The T-Piece. 'A' is the inspiratory limb of oxygen tubing. 'B' is the T-Piece. 'D' is the endotracheal tube. 'C' is the extra piece of tubing on the exhalation side that prevents the patient from breathing in room air.

It provides no ventilatory support; only an oxygen/air mixture. The patient is typically left on this setup for 30 minutes and then assessed. At the end of 30 minutes, the RT will measure RR and also Vt, with a device known as a Wright respirometer, which is attached to the end of the endotracheal tube. From these measurements, an index known as the rapid shallow breathing index (RSBI) can be calculated. The RSBI is calculated as RR/Vt in liters. For example, if RR = 20 and Vt is 500, then RSBI is 20/0.5 = 40. It has been found that an RSBI < 105 predicts that the patient can be extubated successfully[6]. Essentially, a low RSBI means the patient is taking slow and deep breaths, which is good. Fast and small breaths generally mean the patient is quite weak and still needs the ventilator. It should also be noted, that since you are running a simulation, one should look at the patient and see how they are doing. If they are comfortable and breathing normally, then likely they can be extubated. If they are tachycardic, tachypnic and appear in distress, then they have failed, regardless of what the RSBI is.

2. <u>Pressure Support Trial</u>

The other way to run the simulation is with a pressure support (PS) trial. Usually the patient is placed on a pressure support of 5-10cm H2O and 5 of PEEP. The idea is that the pressure support will compensate for the resistance in the endotracheal tube and ventilator circuit and will produce a more realistic simulation of someone breathing on their own. As a rough estimate, PS of 10 should be used for a 7.0 endotracheal tube and PS of 5 for an 8.0 tube if one wanted to be precise. However, a PS of 10 and PEEP of 5 is commonly used for any endotracheal tube size, and results have been acceptable with that. The process is similar to a T-Piece trial. After 30 minutes on PS the patient is assessed. If the patient is breathing comfortably, and is not in distress, then generally the patient can be extubated. An RSBI can be calculated here as well. It should be noted that the RSBI cutoff of < 105 was determined on a T-Piece. It is harder to breathe through a T-piece as there is no pressure support or PEEP. As a result, the RSBI should be < 60 to 70 on PS to predict a successful extubation. As a side note, if you place the patient on PS = 0 and PEEP = 0, you have a condition called 'flow-by'. This likely is somewhat harder to breathe through than a T-piece, as you have to factor in the added resistance of the ventilator circuit. Its advantage over T-piece is that you can read off real-time RR and Vt from the ventilator. I don't commonly use this in my practice to liberate patients from the ventilator as it is not clear how much additional work of breathing is added by the ventilator circuit. By the way, one does not need to worry that the patient may 'stop breathing' while on pressure support, as there is an apnea backup setting built into the machine.

At our institution, SBT's are done using Pressure Support. If a patient was intubated for pulmonary edema, occasionally we will use a T-Piece trial here, as the PS/CPAP will decrease preload and afterload and effectively 'treat' the pulmonary edema, potentially causing the patient to look better on the SBT than they would after extubation.

If there is doubt as to whether a patient can be extubated after a 30 minute spontaneous breathing trial, one can extend the trial to 2 hours, or one can get a blood gas to help determine if the patient is extubatable.

If the patient struggles after extubation, occasionally they are placed on Bi-level NIV. Studies have shown that outcomes are not improved if this strategy is attempted, and may actually be worsened[7]. Rescuing someone who is failing after extubation is different than extubating a high risk, eg. COPD patient, directly to Bi-level NIV. In the latter circumstance, outcomes have been found to be improved[8]. If a patient is extubated and starts to fail, consider reintubation over trying to salvage them with NIV.

Once daily SBT's have been found to be equivalent to multiple daily SBT's[9]. Unless you are dealing with a problem likely to have rapid resolution, i.e. pulmonary edema or a drug overdose, generally the SBT is done once daily.

Daily sedation vacations should be performed in most patients in the ICU. Some studies have shown that daily sedation vacations, as opposed to continuous sedation until the physician thinks the patient is ready to liberate from the ventilator, lead to decreased days on the ventilator[10]. Sedation vacations should generally not be performed on patients requiring very high FiO2 and PEEP, as ventilator dyssynchrony and desaturation may result. Also, they should not be performed on patients receiving NM blockade. Patients intubated for stridor or obstructing airway lesions should generally not have a sedation vacation done until the problem is fixed. This is because a self-extubation in this population is potentially fatal. Also, it is reasonable to do sedation vacations without doing an SBT in patients who are clearly not ready to be extubated.

Occasionally, a patient will be intubated due to stridor or other upper airway problem. Extubating these patients can be challenging, as one needs to determine if a patent upper airway is present. Bronchoscopy or laryngoscopy here usually is not very helpful, as the endotracheal tube obscures the vocal cords. A cuff leak test is where the endotracheal tube cuff is deflated entirely. Normally, a significant amount of air will escape past the cuff during a delivered breath from the ventilator when the cuff is deflated. If there is a significant amount of upper airway swelling or vocal cord edema, then there is no space around the endotracheal tube for the air to pass, and no cuff leak will be present. This tells you that there may be a problem. To determine if a cuff leak is present, one listens carefully after the endotracheal tube cuff is deflated. This is the qualitative technique, and it takes some experience to ascertain if a significant amount of leak is present, versus only a very small leak. One can also use a quantitative method by assessing the difference between the set Vt on the ventilator and the measured returned volume. The difference between the two is the amount of air that leaked out past the deflated cuff. Some studies have shown a leak volume of >110cc's on a volume cycled ventilator mode suggests enough airway patency for the patient to be extubated[11]. Pressure support mode generally should not be used to determine if a cuff leak is present, as there may not be enough pressure to determine if a leak exists. A cuff leak test should be performed prior to extubation in all patients suspected of having an upper airway problem. However, it is not routinely checked in patients not suspected of having an upper airway problem.

Sometimes, a patient will develop post-extubation stridor caused by the intubation process itself, or by the endotracheal tube irritating the vocal cords, causing glottic or subglottic edema. If it is only mild, and the patient is not in respiratory distress, racemic epinephrine nebulizer and steroids can be given, and the patient observed. If it is severe, and the patient is dyspneic and struggling, then the patient should be reintubated. Decadron 6 mg q6h or equivalent for 24 hours is given. The cuff leak test is then performed. If a good leak is present, the patient can be extubated safely. If no leak is present, wait another day and recheck for a cuff leak. If after several days no leak is found, consider a tracheostomy.

It is generally considered acceptable to have a 10% reintubation rate. If a surgeon doing appendectomies, for example, found acute appendicitis 100% of the time they operated, this means they are missing many cases of appendicitis. Similarly, if one had a 100% success rate of extubation, this likely means one is not extubating patients in a timely fashion.

7. Advanced Oxygenation Techniques

When confronted with a patient who is difficult to oxygenate despite high FiO2 and PEEP, a few techniques can be employed.

<u>Prone Ventilation</u>

The PROSEVA trial[12] established prone ventilation as a mortality-reducing intervention in ARDS. Prone ventilation improves oxygenation via a few mechanisms. Firstly, it takes the weight of the heart off of the lung, thereby improving aeration of the part of the lung that was previously compressed by the heart. Also, atelectasis and secretion accumulation are gravity dependent, and the base of the lung in the supine position suffers most from this. Proning the patient allows gravity dependent blood flow to pass through the less atelectatic anterior lung, thereby improving oxygenation. While the patient is proned, the posterior lung has a chance to open up and aerate better, so when placed back in the supine position, many times the oxygenation remains improved.

The PROSEVA protocol included lung-injured patients with an FiO2 of >/= 60% and PEEP of >/= 5, with a P/F ratio of <150 on those settings. The patients were placed prone for 16 hours, and supine for 8 hours. They underwent an average of 4 proning sessions, and with this, a mortality benefit was realized. I think it is important to aggressively decrease FiO2 and possibly PEEP as able while prone, in order to maximize benefit from this strategy. Decreasing FiO2 and PEEP would hopefully decrease oxygen toxicity and plateau pressures.

Of note, at our institution, we continue to feed patients while prone, albeit at a lower rate, i.e., 20cc/hr. Otherwise, trying to administer all the caloric requirements of the patient in 8 hours is challenging.

Nitric Oxide

Nitric Oxide (NO) is an inhaled pulmonary vasodilator that can be used to improve oxygenation in the lung-injured patient. Commonly, it is administered at a dose of between 5-40 ppm. Trials have shown NO to improve oxygenation, but as of yet, none has shown a mortality benefit. Side effects include methemoglobinemia.

ECMO

ECMO stands for extracorporeal membrane oxygenation. Essentially, a long, large bore dialysis-type catheter is placed into the jugular vein, and blood is run from the patient through the ECMO machine and then back into the patient. The oxygenator in the ECMO unit oxygenates the blood and also removes CO_2. This modality is generally reserved for patients failing all other attempts to oxygenate the patient. Studies have shown that early ECMO v late (salvage) ECMO have similar outcomes[13]. As ECMO has quite a high resource utilization, and carries significant morbidity, in our institutions it is used in a salvage fashion. Appropriate candidates may be selected based on the following criteria:

a) P/F ratio of <80 on FiO_2 >90% for more than 6 hours.
b) Ph <7.25 and PCO_2 >60 despite a RR of 36 for more than 6 hours. (This criterion is not commonly used at our institution).
c) Time on ventilator < 7 days.
d) Lack of significant comorbidities including advanced age.

Neuromuscular Blockade

NM blockade can help to oxygenate patients. It accomplishes this mostly by improving ventilator synchrony, and possibly by decreasing lung inflammation[14]. Generally speaking, this should be reserved for patients requiring high FiO_2 and PEEP, as an increased incidence of neuromuscular weakness has been linked to NM blockade. The ACURASYS trial[15] found an improved mortality for severe ARDS patients who received 48 hours of NM blockade early in the disease course. However, the ROSE study,[16] performed later, did not find any significant benefit. It is generally accepted that NM blockade will improve oxygenation, but its effect on mortality has been found to be inconsistent.

8. Sedatives for Mechanical Ventilation

Sedation is important for the mechanically ventilated patient, as being intubated is inherently uncomfortable and anxiety provoking. Here we will discuss common sedatives used for this purpose.

Propofol is probably the most common sedative for mechanical ventilation used in our ICU. It has rapid onset, and wears off 15 minutes after the drug is discontinued. Its action is predominantly via GABA receptors. It is in a lipid emulsion, and can raise plasma triglyceride levels. If used for more than a few days, daily triglyceride levels should be checked, and the drug should be stopped if levels are >500, as there is a risk of pancreatitis with very high triglyceride levels. Side effects include hypotension and bradycardia. 'Propofol infusion syndrome' is a condition characterized by shock, bradycardia, acidosis, rhabdomyolysis and renal failure. It is a rare, but potentially fatal complication, and tends to occur in patients on high doses of propofol for a prolonged duration. Propofol may also turn urine green at high infusion rates. However, this is a benign finding and does not require intervention. Propofol has a mild bronchodilator effect.

Benzodiazepines such as midazolam and lorazepam are useful and common sedatives in the ICU. They have strong anxiolytic properties. Common infusion rates are 1-10 mg/hr. These drugs can also be used as an IV push. Side effects include prolonged residual sedation, as these drugs have a large volume of distribution and tend to be absorbed by fat tissue. This tends to be a bigger problem in obese patients. Lorazepam is dispensed in a propylene glycol diluent. Propylene glycol toxicity can occasionally occur with high infusion rates. This presents as a lactic acidosis. Patients on high infusion rates should have a daily serum osmolarity checked, and if it is elevated, lorazepam should be replaced with another sedative. Also, benzodiazepines have been associated with an increased incidence of delirium[17].

Fentanyl is useful as a sedative in intubated patients. Common infusion rates are 25-150 mcg/hr. It is a synthetic opioid, and hence can be given to patients with a morphine allergy, as there is no cross reactivity between the two drugs. Side effects can be constipation, and rarely, chest wall rigidity. Combining fentanyl with benzodiazepines works well, as there is a combination of anxiolysis and analgesia. Sedative effects of fentanyl are short lived, and it generally wears off after an hour.

Ketamine infusion has recently gained popularity for sedation of ventilated patients. It causes a dissociative anesthesia similar to a 'trance'. It is unique in that it generally does not cause hypotension. It also does not impair airway reflexes or cause respiratory depression. It has some analgesic effects. Side effects include psychotic emergence reactions and increased oral secretions. Dosing is 0.04 -2.5 mg/kg/hr. Like propofol, it has a mild bronchodilator effect.

Dexmedetomidine (Precedex®) is an alpha-2 adrenergic agonist. It is a good choice for sedation of ventilated patients. It does not impair airway reflexes or cause respiratory depression. This allows practitioners to extubate agitated patients safely while continuing the dexmedetomidine infusion. If one is doing a sedation vacation and the patient becomes agitated, consider starting dexmedetomidine and performing the SBT after the patient relaxes some. Side effects include bradycardia, hypotension, and rarely drug fever.

9. Neuromuscular Blockade

NM blockade can be useful to help ventilate or oxygenate patients. It is important, therefore, to know how to implement and use NM blockade for the ventilated patient in the ICU. Indications for NM blockade include, but are not limited to, the following:

- Severe asthma exacerbations where expiratory time needs to be maximized.
- Abdominal compartment syndrome in order to decrease compartment pressure.
- Severe lung injury with difficult oxygenation.
- Patients with very bad ventilator synchrony in order to minimize self-inflicted lung injury, derecruitment, and barotrauma.

NM blockade paralyzes skeletal muscle. It does not affect cardiac or smooth muscle. Consequently, one can continue to feed patients enterally while on NM blockade. Of note, pupillary function is generally not affected. There are two classes of paralytics that are available: depolarizing and nondepolarizing. Depolarizing agents bind to Ach receptors at the neuromuscular junction and cause sustained and prolonged depolarization, resulting in inhibition of muscle contraction. Nondepolarizing agents competitively inhibit Ach-induced depolarization and myocyte activation and cause paralysis by preventing depolarization. Succinylcholine is the only commonly used paralytic that is depolarizing. It is mainly used for rapid sequence intubation and is not used for sustained paralysis of intubated patients. The nondepolarizing paralytics include cisatracurium, rocuronium and vecuronium. Rocuronium and vecuronium are eliminated by the liver and kidneys, and their effects may be prolonged if dysfunction of those organs is present. Cisatracurium is hydrolyzed by plasma esters and is not dependent on liver or kidney function for elimination. For this reason, it is the main paralytic used at our institution. Regardless of which agent is used, it is administered as a bolus dose followed by a continuous infusion.

All patients who are undergoing NM blockade require sedation. Once someone is paralyzed, it is essentially impossible to tell how well they are sedated, as they are unable to move or respond in any way. Being paralyzed and not sedated is a terrifying situation for the patient and needs to be avoided. Tachycardia and hypertension may be a clue to this condition being present. In order to ascertain the level of sedation of a paralyzed patient, a monitor known as the Bi-spectral index (BIS) monitor® is used. This device measures brain activity and outputs a unitless number known as the Bi-spectral (BIS) index. A BIS index of < 60 correlates with deep sedation, and is the goal for paralyzed patients. Usually, the practitioner sedates the patient to a BIS index of < 60 first, and once that is achieved, NM blockade is commenced.

Monitoring depth of paralysis is done using a train-of-four (TOF) stimulator. This is a peripheral nerve stimulator usually placed on the distal ulnar nerve. Twitches of the thumb are then observed. The TOF stimulator administers 4 sequential electrical impulses. As the depth of paralysis with a nondepolarizing agent increases, the number of times the thumb twitches in response to the 4 impulses diminishes or fades. A nonparalyzed person will yield 4 twitches. An excessively paralyzed patient will yield zero twitches. One aims for 1-2 twitches as a goal for appropriate depth of paralysis.

When paralyzing a patient with severe ARDS, one generally starts off with continuous paralysis for 48 hours. This is mostly due to the findings of the ACURASYS trial[15]. After 48 hours has elapsed, one tries to stop the NM blockade and observe how the patient responds. If lung function remains extremely poor, and the patient continues to require very high FiO2 and PEEP, it is acceptable to continue NM blockade for longer without interruption. Also, if the patient de-recruits, desaturates, or has significant problems with synchrony when they are trialed off the paralytic, one may restart the paralytic as needed. As a general rule, one should try to accomplish appropriate ventilation without a paralytic, and if a paralytic is used, one should try to limit how long it is used for, as NM blockade is a known risk factor for critical illness neuropathy/myopathy.

10. Estimating the Degree of Lung Injury

Estimating the degree of lung injury a patient has is helpful in determining if the patient is improving or worsening day to day, and also helps to determine the patient's readiness for liberation from the ventilator. An estimate of how injured the lung is should be done daily on every patient on a ventilator. The approach to this needs to be quick and practical. Lung injury scoring systems such as the Murray lung injury score exist, but are too cumbersome for bedside use. Four basic parameters need to be looked at and assessed. 1) Lung compliance 2) Airway resistance 3) Efficiency of ventilation and 4) Oxygenation.

Lung compliance, as stated before, is calculated as change in volume / change in pressure. The lower the respiratory system compliance is, the more damaged the lung is. A good way to rapidly check lung compliance is to look at the peak airway pressure. If it is <30, then you know the Pplat is ok because Pplat is always less than Ppeak. This is quick and easy and does not require you to perform an inspiratory pause maneuver. It is inexact, but for general gestalt purposes it will suffice.

Assessing the ability of the lung to oxygenate can help us determine the degree of lung injury as well. A P/F ratio can be easily calculated. A quick and dirty method to estimate the lung's ability to oxygenate blood, is to multiply the FiO2 being delivered by 5. The PO2 of a normal patient will be 5 x the FiO2. For example, a healthy patient breathing room air will have a PO2 of 5 x 21% = 105. If someone with normal lungs is on a ventilator at 100% FiO2, they should have a PO2 of roughly 5 x 100% = 500. If someone is on 100% FiO2 and the resulting PO2 is only 90, then you know the patient has a significant alveolar-arterial gradient (A-a gradient) and severe lung function impairment.

Assessing the relationship between minute ventilation and PCO_2 can tell us how efficiently the patient's lung can ventilate or blow off carbon dioxide. A normal person at rest, breathing room air, will have a minute ventilation of around 4-5 lpm. This results in a PCO_2 of 40. If a patient on a ventilator has a minute ventilation of 15 lpm and a PCO_2 of 40, that tells you the patient has significant dead space, and consequently, an injured lung.

Airway resistance and bronchospasm should be assessed. Auscultating the patient can tell you if wheezing is present, or if a 'silent' lung is present, indicating severe airflow limitation. Here again, looking at the Ppeak tells you a lot very quickly. If the Ppeak is < 30, severe bronchospasm is unlikely to be present. One can quickly look at the flow waveform to rapidly assess if autopeep is present. A more formal measurement of airway resistance as outlined in chapter 4 can be done, but is generally not necessary routinely.

11. Complications of Mechanical Ventilation

Barotrauma and volutrauma refer to injury to the lung due to airway pressure and inflation volume. The manifestations of this are pneumothorax, pneumomediastinum and subcutaneous air. In regards to airway pressures, it is thought that the plateau pressure matters more than the peak pressure. In fact, it is not clear that the peak pressure matters much at all as long as the plateau pressure is acceptable. The ARDSnet study (5) identified a goal of 6 ml/kg as a reasonable inflation volume, after which mortality started to increase incrementally with increasing volume. The reality is, the less one beats up the patient's lung the better. One should try to ventilate the patient with the minimum ventilator settings that get the job done.

Oxygen toxicity refers to toxic injury to the lung due to free radical generation from high FiO2. It is thought that significant risk starts at around an FiO2 of 60%. Manifestations of oxygen toxicity are thought to include tracheitis, lung injury and ARDS. Oxygen toxicity can occur on or off the ventilator. One should keep in mind that the ventilator is delivering oxygen under positive pressure, and therefore can deliver higher levels of oxygen than someone not on positive pressure. We can compare a patient on the ventilator with a mean pressure (Pmean) of 30 on 100% FiO2, with someone receiving 100% O2 at atmospheric pressure using the alveolar gas equation.

$$PAO2 = (Patm - PH2O) \times FiO2 - (PCO2/RQ)$$

Where RQ is the respiratory quotient and is around 0.8, and PH2O is the water vapor pressure and is around 45 mm Hg. PAO2 is the partial pressure of oxygen in the alveolus.

a) Sea level PAO2 on FiO2 100% = (760 – 45) x 1.0 – (40/0.8)
   = 665
b) Pmean of 30 on ventilator set at 100% FiO2. PAO2 = (782 – 45) x 1.0 – (40/0.8) = 687

760 mmHg is the partial pressure of 100% oxygen at atmospheric pressure and 782 is the partial pressure of 100% oxygen in mm hg at 30cm H2O pressure.

It is not clear how much this affects things clinically, but it is worth noting at least as a thought exercise. Of note, as much as we talk about oxygen toxicity and its dangers, clinical evidence of its effect is still lacking.

Vocal cord edema/subglottic stenosis may occur in ventilated patients. Traumatic intubation may increase the likelihood of this. Although common sense would suggest that the longer someone has been intubated, the more likely one would develop vocal cord edema and/or subglottic stenosis, this has not been demonstrated clearly in studies. One generally realizes someone has this problem only AFTER extubating the patient, when stridor and signs of upper airway obstruction are observed. See earlier discussion on cuff leak testing in chapter 6 regarding how to proceed if this complication occurs.

Ventilator associated pneumonia (VAP) is pneumonia that develops after 48 hours on a ventilator. Diagnosis is by detection of fever, leukocytosis, purulent endotracheal secretions, and chest x-ray findings of pneumonia. It is associated with worsened overall outcomes including mortality. Risk factors for VAP include, but are not limited to:

a) Advanced age
b) Underlying lung disease
c) Proton pump inhibitors
d) Prolonged ventilation
e) Frequent ventilator circuit changes

Strategies to reduce VAP include:

a) Daily sedation vacations, as this decreases total days on the ventilator
b) Minimize sedation
c) Use noninvasive ventilation when able
d) Use an endotracheal tube with a subglottic drainage port
e) Head of bed kept at 30 degrees

12. Other Modes of Oxygenation/Ventilation

The nasal cannula is the most commonly used means of delivering oxygen. As a rough guide, for every lpm flow of oxygen through a nasal cannula, the FiO2 increases by 3%. For example, a patient on 2 lpm nasal cannula oxygen would be getting roughly 2 lpm x 3% = 6% + 21% (room air FiO2) = 27% total FiO2. Due to issues of mucosal irritation/dryness/epistaxis, the nasal cannula isn't practical or effective beyond 8-10 lpm.

When contemplating the FiO2 delivered by a simple oxygen device (nasal cannula, face mask, venti mask or nonrebreather) one needs to keep in mind that the FiO2 that we are interested in is the one delivered to the upper airway. The oxygen concentration of 1 lpm nasal cannula measured at the cannula tip is actually 100%. As the patient breathes in, he/she entrains room air, thereby decreasing the FiO2 delivered to the upper airway. If the patient is breathing rapidly, the patient may inhale a 500cc tidal volume in 0.5 seconds. That is equal to a 60 lpm flow rate for each breath. If one is receiving oxygen at 1 lpm from a nasal cannula, one can see that only a small fraction of the inspired gas that is delivered to the upper airway will be from the nasal cannula. Most of it will be room air. CONCEPT: An important point to remember is that the effective FiO2 delivered by a simple oxygen device is INVERSELY proportional to the patient's minute ventilation. This does not apply to CPAP or Bi-level NIV, as that with a good mask seal, it can deliver effectively unlimited flow and close to 100% FiO2.

Facemask oxygen is better at delivering higher FiO2 due to the fact that the gas isn't directed directly into the nares, so mucosal irritation/dryness/epistaxis is less of a concern. Up to 15 lpm can be delivered this way. The mask form factor also has a small amount of a reservoir function that stores the accumulated oxygen when the patient is in between breaths, thereby increasing the FiO2 delivered to the upper airway. A venturi mask (venti mask for short) is a simple mask with a venturi valve fitted at the oxygen inlet. This mask utilizes the Bernoulli principle to allow for a more precise delivery of FiO2. One can select FiO2 in 5% increments depending on which valve/setting is used. As high-speed oxygen passes through the valve, the drop in pressure this creates entrains a specific amount of room air. A venti mask can be titrated to 60% FiO2.

The nonrebreather mask is a facemask oxygen delivery device which utilizes a plastic bag reservoir. When the patient is exhaling, the bag fills with oxygen. When the patient takes the next breath in, the patient receives oxygen from this reservoir, as well as from the continuous stream of oxygen that is being delivered, thereby increasing the total amount of oxygen that can be delivered per breath. Compare this to a simple mask, where during exhalation, the oxygen flowing into the mask is lost to the room instead of being stored. The FiO2 delivered by a nonrebreather is around 70-80%.

Humidified high flow nasal cannula (HHFNC) is a more recent oxygen delivery device. Trade names include Optiflo® and Vapotherm®. These devices can deliver 60 lpm of 100% oxygen through the cannula. The reason this high flow is possible, is through the use of heated humidification. If one tried to deliver this much flow without heat and humidity, mucosal dryness/irritation/epistaxis would ensue. The effect of delivering this very high flow rate is the ability to deliver nearly 100% FiO2. Also, due to the very high flow, there is washout of CO2 from the upper airway. This has the effect of decreasing dead space. This can contribute to increased ventilatory efficiency, decreased work of breathing, and possibly decreased PCO2. So, in addition to improving oxygenation, there is some effect of improving ventilation, although it is not as effective as Bi-level NIV in this regard. The high flow rate also delivers some amount of PEEP. It is thought that for every 10 lpm flow, 0.5cm of PEEP is generated.

One additional advantage of HHFNC is that the patient can eat while on this device.

Noninvasive positive pressure ventilation (CPAP or Bi-level NIV) is able to deliver nearly 100% effective FiO2. The unit can deliver effectively unlimited flow. As there is a sealed mask interface, room air entrainment is minimized. In practice, a port on the CPAP/NIV interface is left open for exhalation, so a small amount of entrainment will occur through this. CPAP is one fixed pressure both during inhalation and exhalation. Bi-level NIV delivers a higher pressure during inhalation (inspiratory positive airway pressure or 'IPAP'), and a lower pressure during exhalation (expiratory positive airway pressure or 'EPAP'). This increase in pressure during inhalation helps to ventilate the patient, hence its common use in COPD exacerbations. The delta between the IPAP and the EPAP determines how much ventilatory support is being given. The higher the delta, the more the support. As a teaching point, the convention for NIV is that the IPAP pressure equals the actual measured peak pressure. On a ventilator set to pressure support, which is a similar setting to Bi- level NIV, the pressure support is the pressure *above* the PEEP setting. Therefore, a Bi-level NIV set at 10/5 would have a Ppeak of 10cm H2O whereas a ventilator set at PS 10/5 would have a Ppeak of 15cm H2O. Bi-level NIV is the highest level of respiratory support of all the noninvasive methods.

13. Practical Respiratory Physiology

In this chapter we will discuss practical points of respiratory physiology that have real world bedside implications.

The Oxygen Dissociation Curve

The oxygen dissociation curve is important, as it many times explains the common discrepancy between the oxygen saturation and the PO2 (Fig 13). Various factors can impact the affinity of hemoglobin for oxygen. If something increases the affinity of hemoglobin for oxygen, then the oxygen dissociation curve is shifted leftward. This left-shifted curve will demonstrate a higher oxygen saturation for any given PO2. Conversely, anything that causes hemoglobin's affinity for oxygen to decrease, will shift the curve to the right. A right-shifted curve would show a lower oxygen saturation for any given PO2. In the ICU, the most common parameters that alter the affinity of hemoglobin for oxygen, and hence the oxygen dissociation curve, are pH and temperature. When a patient is undergoing therapeutic hypothermia, the oxygen saturation will appear *higher* than the PO2 on the blood gas would suggest. Acidosis will make the oxygen saturation appear *lower* than what would be expected. The next time an acidotic patient on a ventilator is receiving a push of IV bicarbonate, stand at the bedside and watch what happens. You will likely see the oxygen saturation rise immediately, in real time. A helpful tip to remember the relationship between PO2 and oxygen saturation is the 30-60-90 rule. A PO2 of 30 yields an O2 saturation of around 60%, and a PO2 of 60 yields an O2 saturation of around 90%. Also, if the O2 saturation is 100%, generally the PO2 will be >/= to 100.

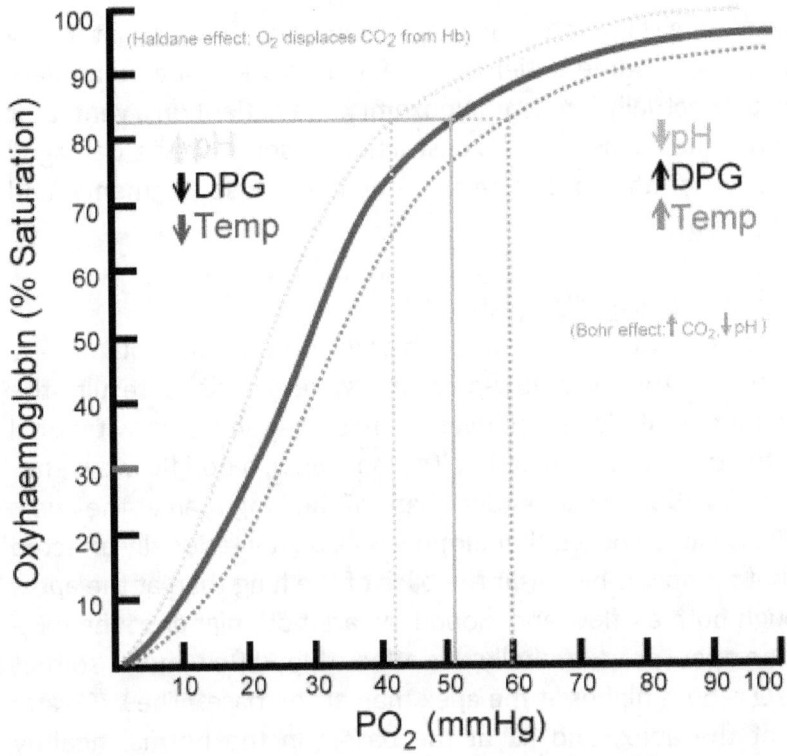

Figure 13. The oxygen dissociation curve. Hypothermia and alkalosis will increase the affinity of hemoglobin for oxygen and shift the curve leftward.

Hypoxic Vasoconstriction

An interesting adaptive response takes place in the lung when alveolar hypoxia occurs. The pulmonary arterioles in the region of the poorly oxygenated alveoli vasoconstrict and limit blood flow to that segment of lung. This reduces pulmonary shunt and limits the impact of the impaired lung unit on systemic oxygenation. This physiologic response would be at play, for example, in someone with pneumonia. The consolidated lung segments would have alveolar hypoxia, and consequently those lung segments would vasoconstrict so that blood flow through the damaged lung is limited. The practical import of this is that it may explain why, in some patients, the administration of a pulmonary vasodilator actually worsens hypoxemia. If a patient on a ventilator with ARDS has hypoxic vasoconstriction in some of the damaged lung, adding inhaled NO may vasodilate those segments and worsen shunt.

West Lung Zones and V/Q ratio

The right heart pumps blood through the pulmonary circulation. This is a low-pressure system. As a result, the pulmonary circulation is relatively more susceptible to gravitational flow effects. In the upright, healthy individual, blood flow is higher in the gravitationally dependent base of the lung than at the apex. Also, it should be noted that air flow is also gravitationally affected and that air flow is higher at the base of the lung than at the apex. Although both air flow and blood flow are both higher at the base than the apex, proportionally this affects blood flow more, so that the V/Q ratio is higher at the apex than at the base. The V/Q ratio is >1 at the apex, and <1 at the base. In the normal healthy individual, the V/Q ratios both at the apex and base are close to 1 resulting in minimal dead space or shunt. In the diseased lung, however, the V/Q ratios may be much greater or less than one resulting in significant dead space and shunt. A V/Q ratio >> 1 results in dead space and a V/Q ratio << 1 produces shunt.

The West lung zones describe regional variations in blood flow and pressure due to this gravitational effect (Fig 14). West zone 1 occurs at the lung apex. Here the capillary pressure is very low and is actually exceeded by the alveolar pressure. Because the alveolar pressure is higher than the capillary pressure, the capillary is occluded and no blood flow takes place here. This zone represents physiologic dead space and has a V/Q ratio >>1. In the normal healthy person, there is little to none of this zone present. West zone 3 describes what occurs at the base of the lung. Here, hydrostatic pressure is the greatest, and alveolar pressure is

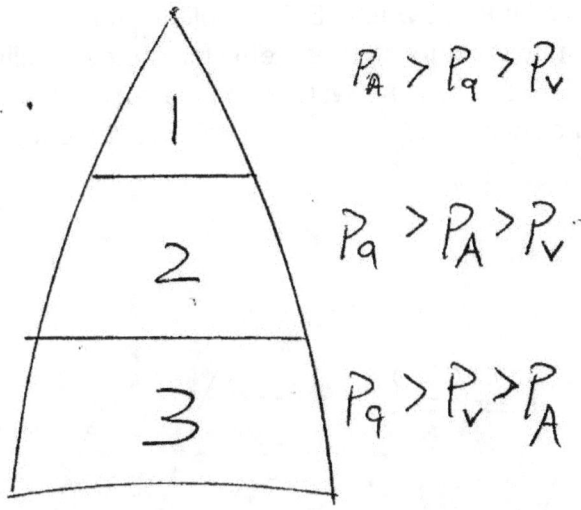

Figure 14. West zones of the lung. Zones are labeled 1,2 and 3. PA = alveolar pressure. Pa = arteriolar pressure. Pv = venous pressure.

eclipsed by both arteriolar and venous pressure. Blood flow is highest in this region resulting in the lowest V/Q ratio of any of the zones. West zone 2 is in the middle portion of the lung. Here, the alveolar pressure is less than the arteriolar pressure, but greater than the venous pressure. Blood flow in this region of the lung is dependent on the difference between the arteriolar and alveolar pressures and independent of the venous pressure. Flow here is somewhat pulsatile and occurs mostly in systole. This lung region will have a V/Q ratio in between zone 1 and zone 3.

What is the clinical importance of knowing about West lung zones and V/Q ratios? It helps us understand some of the effects of PEEP on the lung. PEEP increase alveolar pressure (PA). This converts some of lung zone 3 into lung zone 2. It also converts some of lung zone 2 into lung zone 1. The net effect is to increase zone 1 and decrease zone 3 (Fig 15). This creates more dead space and less shunt. We see the clinical results of this in a higher PO2 and also a slightly higher PCO2 when PEEP is applied. Interestingly, hypovolemia can mimic some of these effects. A lower filling pressure of the RV will decrease RV systolic and diastolic pressures and will create more zone 1 and less zone 3 similar to the effect of PEEP.

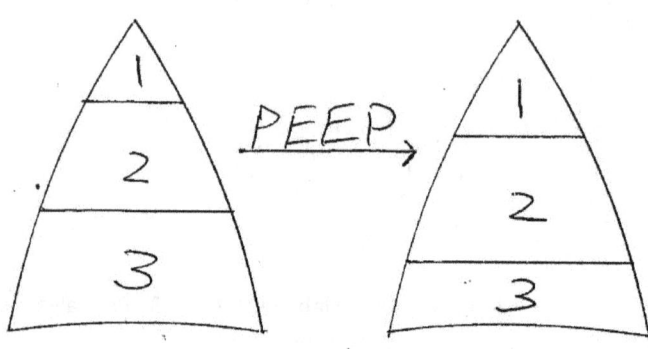

Figure 15. The application of PEEP increases West zone 1 and decreases zone 3.

The Pulmonary Compliance Curve

The pressure-volume curve of the respiratory system is derived by applying a known pressure to the respiratory system and measuring the change in volume that results from the added pressure. If one plots the lung volumes that result from incrementally increasing pressures, one will generate a curve as in figure 16. The curve represented here is a bit of an oversimplification, as the real curve differs between inspiration and expiration; a concept known as *hysteresis* which is beyond the scope of this book. Starting at the residual volume, we see that at low volumes, the system is poorly compliant. This is due to surface tension in the lung. The system then reaches a lower inflection point (LIP), after which the system is very compliant. At high lung

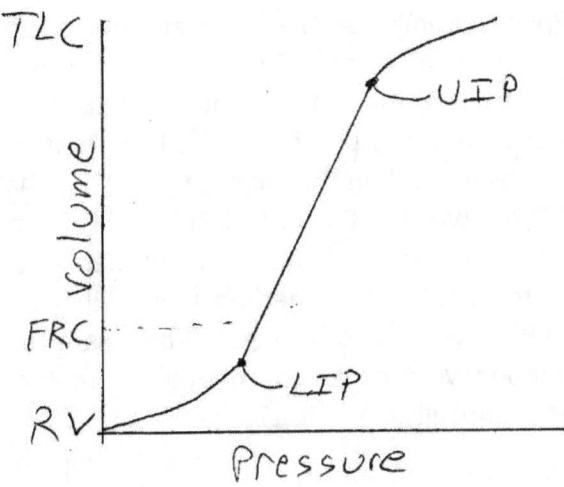

Figure 16. The pressure-volume curve of the respiratory system. LIP = lower inflection point. UIP = upper inflection point. RV = residual volume. TLC = total lung capacity. FRC = functional residual capacity and is just above the lower inflection point of the curve.

volumes, the system reaches an upper inflection point (UIP), after which compliance again becomes poor. This is due to mechanical restriction of the chest wall. On the compliant portion of the curve, in between the upper and lower inflection points, we see that the curve is relatively linear and has a constant slope. How is this information helpful to us clinically? We can use this curve to help us titrate PEEP. Generally, we want the tidal volume to be delivered somewhere along the compliant portion of the curve. Because the compliant portion of the curve is linear and has a constant slope, a given Vt on this portion of the curve will generate the same change in pressure in the system regardless of where it is on that part of the curve. As we increase PEEP, FRC rises until it approaches the UIP. As long as the VT is being delivered somewhere along the compliant portion of the curve and below the UIP, the Ppeak and Pplat will increase the same amount as the increase in PEEP. That is, if you increase PEEP by two, for example, the Ppeak and Pplat will also increase by two. Once the PEEP is set so high that the Vt is delivered at a point past the UIP, then the Ppeak and Pplat will rise by *more* than the increase in PEEP. That is, if you increase PEEP by two, the Ppeak and Pplat will rise by perhaps five. Once you have reached this point, probably you should back down on the PEEP. This method may help us in knowing the maximum PEEP we should deliver, but be aware that the injured lung may not behave as expected, and that this method has not been validated empirically. See Fig 17.

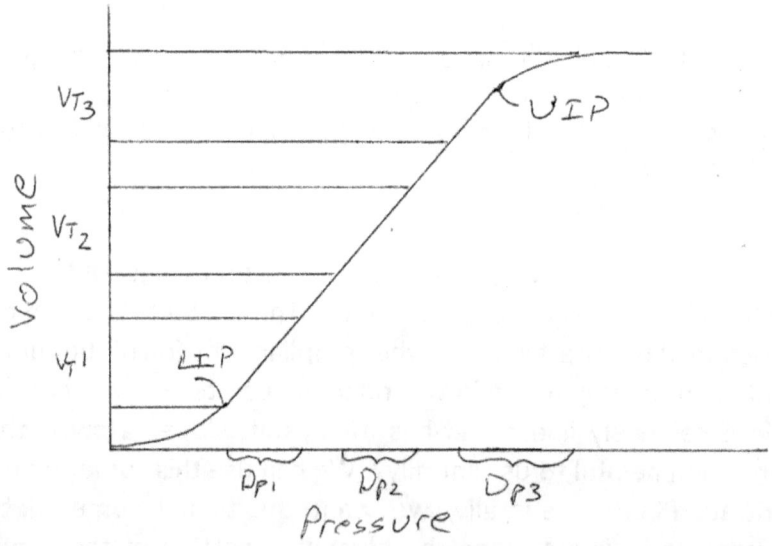

Figure 17. Three identical tidal volumes delivered at three different levels of PEEP. Vt1 and Vt2 generate the same Dp because they are both delivered along the compliant portion of the curve. Vt3 generates a higher Dp because part of it is delivered past the upper inflection point (UIP) of the curve.

14. Illustrative Cases

Case 1

A 63-year-old male presents to the emergency room with shortness of breath. This started 2 days ago and has progressed. The patient reports a dry cough, but no chest pain or fevers. In the ED, he is noted to be in distress due to shortness of breath. A brief trial of Bi-level NIV is initiated, but due to persistent distress and hypoxemia he is intubated. He has a history of asthma and congestive heart failure. His ventilator settings are: AC-VC 12, Vt 500, FiO2 100% and PEEP of 5. Flow pattern is square wave at a rate of 60 lpm. The ventilator graphics are shown below.

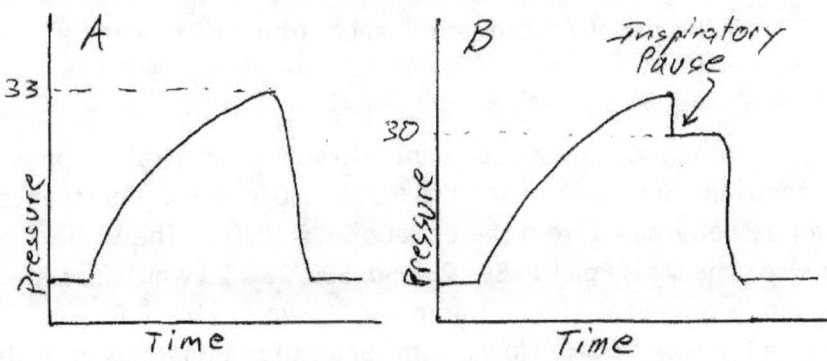

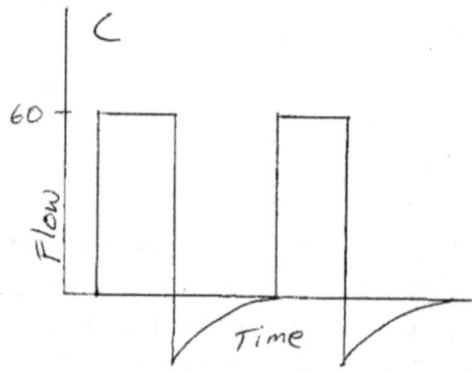

Questions:

1) What is the patient's plateau pressure?
2) What is the respiratory system compliance?
3) What is the airway resistance?
4) Is this patient's respiratory failure from CHF or asthma?

Ventilator graphic 'B' demonstrates an inspiratory pause maneuver. Here we can see the Pplat is 30cm H2O. Compliance can be determined from the equation C = Vt/Dp. The Vt here is 500cc. The Dp is Pplat-PEEP= 25. So, 500/25 = 20 which indicates a poorly compliant lung. From panel 'A' we see the Ppeak is 33. Raw = (Ppeak – Pplat) / Flow in lpm. Since the ventilator is set with a square flow pattern and 60 lpm flow, the denominator becomes one, and this equation becomes: Raw = Ppeak-Pplat = 33 – 30 = 3. This is a normal Raw. Also, from panel 'C', we can see there is no autopeep present, as the flow returns to zero after the breath. The combination of low compliance, normal airway resistance, and no autopeep, suggests this patient's respiratory failure is likely to be from CHF/pulmonary edema rather than asthma.

Case 2

A 34-year-old male with a history of asthma presents to the emergency department with shortness of breath. He is intubated in the ED using rapid sequence intubation. You see the patient in the ED while he is still under the effects of a paralytic. The ventilator settings are the following: AC-VC 24, Vt 450, FiO2 100, PEEP of 5. Flow pattern is square wave set at 60 lpm. Vital signs are: BP 80/40, Temp = 37, HR = 120, RR = 24, O2 saturation = 100%. ABG demonstrates pH = 7.35, PCO2 = 46, PO2 = 355. Ventilator graphics are shown below.

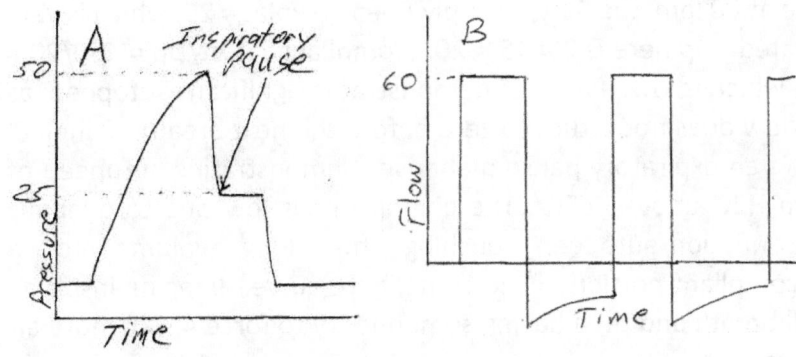

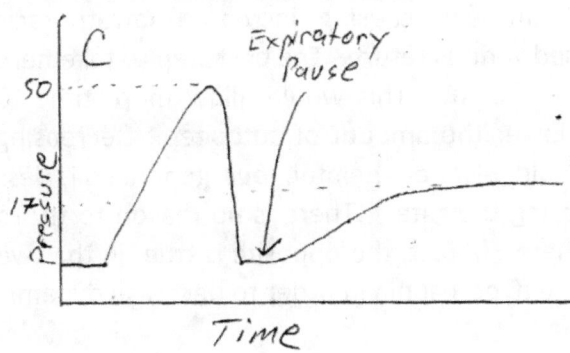

Questions:

1) What is Pplat, Ppeak, Raw and system compliance?
2) What is the best thing to do here?
   a. Increase RR to normalize PCO2
   b. Decrease Vt
   c. Decrease RR
   d. Start norepinephrine

From panel 'A' we can see that Ppeak is 50 which is very high. Pplat is 25, as can be seen from the inspiratory pause maneuver displayed in panel 'A'. Since the flow is set as a square wave at 60 lpm, the Raw is simply Ppeak – Pplat = 25, which is very elevated. Dp here is 25 – 5 = 20. Compliance is Vt/Dp = 450/20 = 22.5 which is low. Panel 'B' demonstrates significant autopeep, as the flow does not return to zero before the next breath. Panel 'C' shows an expiratory pause maneuver demonstrating autopeep of 12cm H2O above PEEP. The compliance is low due to dynamic hyperinflation/autopeep pushing the lung volume to a noncompliant portion of the compliance curve. Imagine inspiring a full breath and then having someone try to force 450cc more air into your lung. It would take a significant amount of pressure to do this. A similar phenomenon occurs when severe autopeep is present. The patient's vital signs demonstrate hypotension. This is very likely due to autopeep causing increased intrathoracic pressure and decreased venous return. The best step to take here would be to decrease the RR. This would allow more time to exhale, and thereby lower the amount of autopeep. Decreasing the tidal volume would also be helpful, but generally is less effective than decreasing the rate. There is no reason to try to normalize the PCO2 here. In fact, the opposite is true, in that we would allow permissive hypercapnia in order to decrease dynamic hyperinflation.

Case 3

A 45-year-old male with a history of asthma, presents to the emergency department with a severe asthma attack. Due to severe distress in the ED, he gets intubated. On ventilator day 3 in the ICU, his condition has improved, and the plan is to do a spontaneous breathing trial. Current ventilator settings are as follows: AC-VC 12, Vt 450, FiO2 40%, PEEP of 5. Flow is a square wave set at 60 lpm. Ventilator graphics on these settings are shown below.

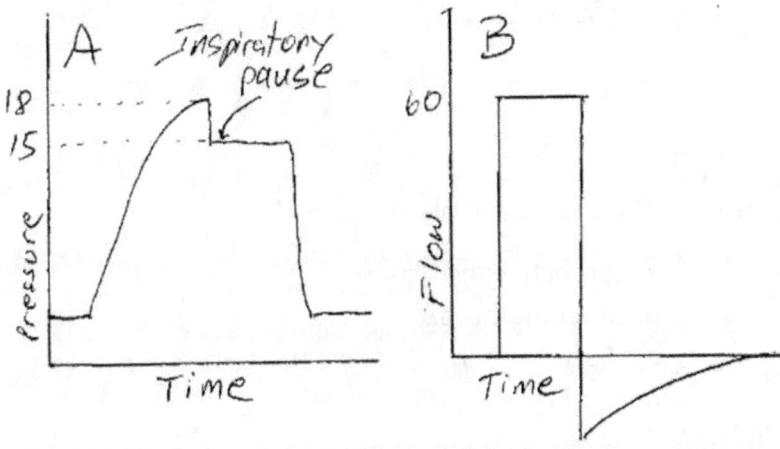

The nurse calls you urgently and states the ventilator alarm is going off and the patient's oxygen saturation is dropping. The following ventilator graphics are now apparent.

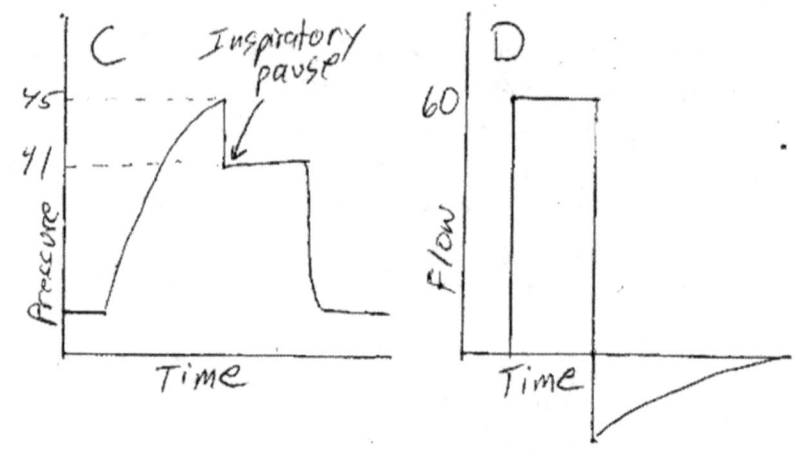

Question: What has taken place?

    a. Bronchoconstriction
    b. Pneumothorax
    c. Secretions in ETT
    d. Cuff leak/rupture

    Comparing ventilator graphics before and after the ventilator starts alarming, we see an acute rise in both the Ppeak and Pplat. They are now 45 and 41 respectively, up from 18 and 15. Raw measured post-alarm, with a square wave set to 60 lpm, is simplified to just Ppeak – Pplat = 4 which is normal. Compliance post-alarm is Vt/Dp = 450 / 36 = 12.5 which is very low. Pre-alarm compliance was 450 / 10 = 45 which was much better. No autopeep is present either before or after the alarm, as can be seen in panels 'B' and 'D', showing no residual flow at the end of the breath. So, whatever occurred decreased compliance, but did not increase Raw. Bronchoconstriction and secretions in the ETT would both increase Raw, so they are unlikely culprits. A blown ETT cuff would decrease Ppeak, making this choice unlikely. The most likely of the choices given here is pneumothorax, which would increase Ppeak and decrease system compliance without increasing Raw.

Case 4

A 55-year-old female presents to the emergency room with a 3-day history of fever, cough and dyspnea. Due to severe respiratory distress and hypoxemia, she is intubated and paralyzed in the ED. Initial ventilator settings are: AC-VC 26, Vt 400, FiO2 100%, PEEP of 10. Initial ABG shows pH = 7.28, PCO2 = 56, PO2 = 110. She is 60 kg ideal body weight. Chest x-ray reveals diffuse bilateral infiltrates. The emergency medicine resident calls you and suggests increasing the RR to help improve the pH. The following ventilator graphics are noted.

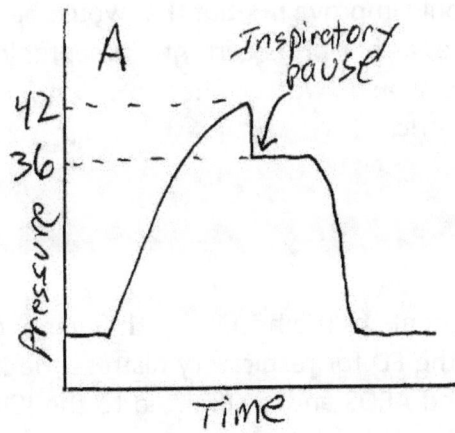

Question: What is the best adjustment to make here?

   a. Increase PEEP
   b. Increase respiratory rate
   c. Decrease respiratory rate
   d. Decrease tidal volume

It is likely this patient has pneumonia with ARDS. The following calculations can be made. Panel 'A' demonstrates an inspiratory pause maneuver resulting in a Pplat of 36. Driving pressure (Dp) = Pplat – PEEP = 36 – 10 = 26. System compliance = Vt/Dp = 400/26 = 15 which is low, indicating a stiff lung. Per ARDSnet, goal Vt is 6cc/kg. The patient's ideal body weight is given as 60 kg. 60 x 6 = 360cc goal Vt. We are above goal for Vt, Dp and Pplat. The best thing to do here would be to decrease the tidal volume and allow permissive hypercapnia. Increasing PEEP here may increase PO2, but oxygenation is currently acceptable. Increasing respiratory rate would improve pH, but that would be a meaningless intervention here, as her pH is currently acceptable. Decreasing respiratory rate would worsen her pH without improving any other useful metric.

Case 5

A 60 year old male presents to the hospital with fever and dyspnea. He is intubated in the ED for respiratory distress. He is diagnosed with pneumonia and ARDS and is admitted to the ICU under your care. Due to difficulty oxygenating the patient, he is administered NM blockade. On day two of his ICU stay, you are rounding in the ICU and note his ventilator settings to be: AC-VC 20, Vt 400, FiO2 60%, PEEP of 8. The flow setting is square wave at 60 lpm. Vital signs are: BP 120/60, T = 37, HR = 90, RR = 20, O2 saturation = 100%. ABG demonstrates pH = 7.39, PCO2 = 41, PO2 = 109. Feeling things look stable, you go to get lunch. While eating, the nurse pages you and states the patient has become tachycardic and has begun to desaturate. After running up to the bedside, you notice the following vital signs: BP 80/50, T = 36, HR = 120, RR = 20, O2 saturation = 81%. An ABG is drawn and demonstrates: pH = 7.20, PCO2 = 70, PO2 = 48. The ventilator graphics are shown below. Panel 'A' is pressure-time pre-event. Panel 'B' is pressure-time post-event. Panel 'C' is the flow graphic post-event.

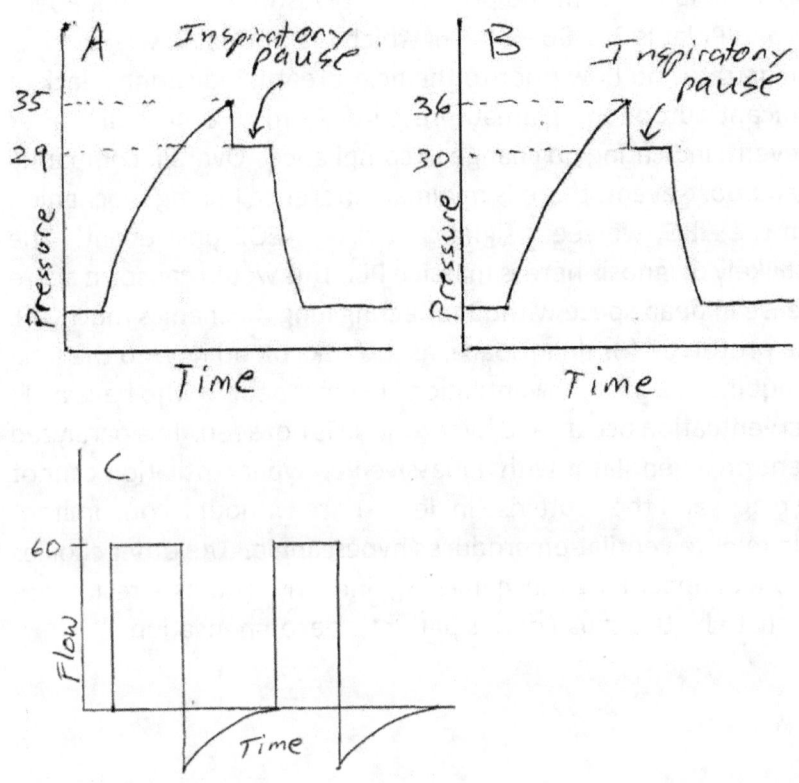

Question: What has taken place here?

    a) Pneumothorax
    b) Bronchospasm
    c) Massive PE
    d) Mucus plug in ET tube

Ppeak is similar before and after the event. Raw is simplified to Ppeak – Pplat, as the flow setting here is a square wave at 60 lpm. From the post-event pressure time curve, Ppeak is 36 and Pplat is 30. 36 – 30 = 6, which is a normal Raw. Panel 'C' demonstrates no flow prior to the next breath, indicating a lack of significant autopeep. Plateau pressure is similar before and after the event, indicating no change in compliance. Overall, comparing pre and post-event, there is minimal difference in lung mechanics. From the ABG, we see a significant rise in CO2 post-event. The most likely diagnosis here is massive PE. This would cause an acute increase in dead space without affecting lung mechanics much. PE is the prototype for dead space, as it blocks blood flow to the lung without interfering with ventilation. In most people who have a PE, hyperventilation occurs and hypercapnia is not seen. In a paralyzed patient on a ventilator with a massive PE, hyperventilation cannot take place, and the acute rise in dead space without a concomitant rise in minute ventilation produces hypercapnia. The other choices would all impact lung mechanics significantly, and as a result, are unlikely to be the cause of this patient's decompensation.

15. Acid Base Chart

Included here is an acid base chart. I have yet to be able to work this out in my head, and I carry a copy of this with me at all times when rounding. I suggest cutting this chart out and laminating it.

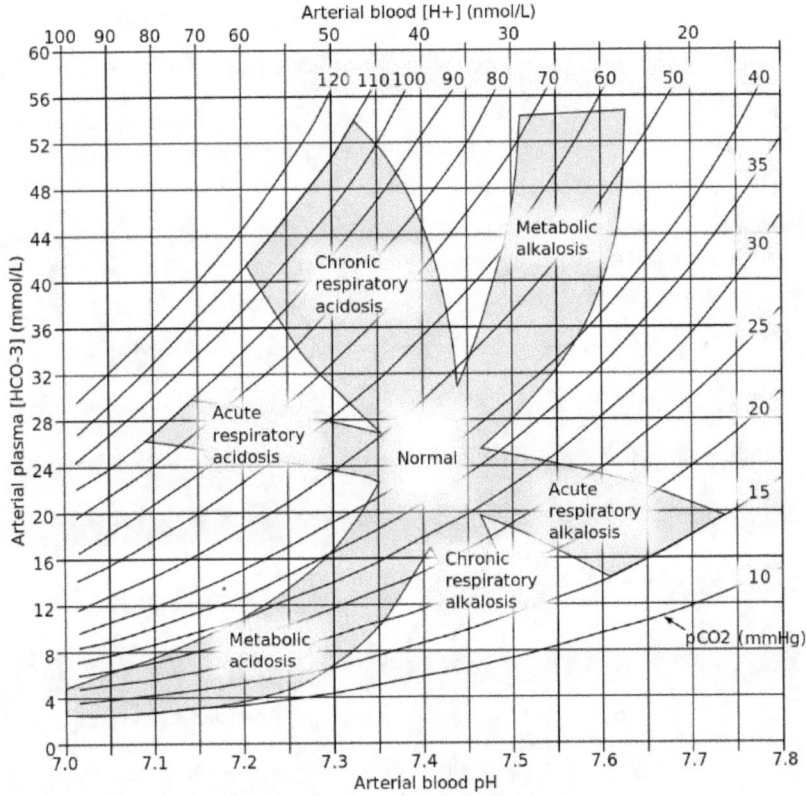

Illustration by HA Finn

Bibliography

1. N Engl J Med 2004; 351:327-336
2. Critical Care V8, 2004:P44
3. Crit Care Med 2017; 45(5):843-850
4. Intensive Care Med 2012; 38(10):1731-2
5. N Engl J Med 2000; 342(18):1301
6. N Engl J Med 1991; 324(21):1445
7. N Engl J Med 2004; 350:2452-2460
8. Am J Resp Crit Care Med 2006; 15; 173(2):164-70
9. N Engl J Med 1995; 332:345-350
10. N Engl J Med 2000; 342:1471-1477
11. Chest 1996; 110(4):1035
12. N Engl J Med 2013; 368:2159-2168
13. N Engl J Med 2018; 378:1965-1975
14. Crit Care Med 2006; 34(11):2749-2757
15. N Engl J Med 2010; 363:1107-1116
16. N Engl J Med 2019; 380:1997-2008
17. Intensive Care Med 2015; 41(12):2130-7

About the Author

Dr. Kutty is a practicing pulmonologist in the Chicagoland area. He lives with his wife Nazneen, children Kabir and Amirah, and cat Max.

www.ingramcontent.com/pod-product-compliance
Lightning Source LLC
Chambersburg PA
CBHW050249220526
45465CB00002B/614